American Medical Association

Physicians dedicated to the health of America

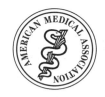

State Medical Licensure Requirements and Statistics

2003

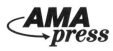

State Medical Licensure Requirements and Statistics

Additional copies of this book may be ordered by calling 800 621-8335. Secure online orders can be taken at www.ama-assn.org/go/catalog. Mention product number OP399002

Comments or inquiries
Fred Donini-Lenhoff, Editor
Medical Education Products
American Medical Association
515 North State Street
Chicago, IL 60610
312 464-5333
312 464-5830 Fax
E-mail: fred_lenhoff@ama-assn.org
www.ama-assn.org/go/licensure

OP399002
ISBN: 1-57947-297-4
BP15:02-P-019:8/02

Foreword

State Medical Licensure Requirements and Statistics 2003 presents current information and statistics on medical licensure in the United States and possessions. Data were obtained from a number of sources, including state boards of medical examiners, the Federation of State Medical Boards, National Board of Medical Examiners, Educational Commission for Foreign Medical Graduates, and the United States Medical Licensing Examination Secretariat.

Licensure data and policies in this publication were compiled from the AMA's 2002 Medical Licensure Survey, which was sent in April 2002 to all 54 allopathic and 13 osteopathic boards of medical examiners in the United States. Although every effort was made to collect and record accurate data for each board, users of this book should note that the boards meet frequently and, as a result, their licensure and examination policies are modified regularly. It is therefore recommended that the state licensing boards (see Appendixes A and B) be contacted for the most up-to-date information.

For more information . . .

The AMA offers Internet information on medical licensure through its Medical Licensure Online Web site (www.ama-assn.org/go/licensure). The site includes information from this book and *Licensing and Credentialing: What Physicians Need to Know*, as well as links to state and national licensing organizations and selected articles on licensure from *American Medical News*.

Also available via the AMA Web site is information on physician-related data resources of the AMA, available at www.ama-assn.org/ama/pub/category/2670.html.

Acknowledgments

The editors would like to thank the personnel of the state medical and osteopathic licensing agencies who provided statistics and licensing requirements for this publication. Special thanks to Randal Manning, executive director of the Maine Board of Licensure in Medicine, for his suggested enhancements to Table 13.

Acknowledgments are also due to the following individuals and organizations for their assistance with updating copy and writing articles:

- Accreditation Council for Graduate Medical Education
  David C. Leach, MD, Executive Director
- American Board of Medical Specialties
  Stephen H. Miller, MD, MPH, Executive Vice President
  Alexis Rodgers, Operations Manager
- Robert D. Aronson, Esquire, author of "Immigration Overview for International Medical Graduates"
- Department of the Air Force
  Sharon R. Ahrari, Lieutenant Colonel, USAF, NC, Chief, Credentialing and Privileging Policy
  Catherine E. Biersack, Colonel (S), USAF, MC Chief, Clinical Quality Management Division
- Department of the Army
  Howard M. Kimes, Colonel, US Army Director, Quality Management Directorate
  Janet L. Wilson, Lieutenant Colonel, US Army, Chief, Regulatory Compliance
- Department of the Navy
  Jan Chandler, Captain, Medical Corps, US Navy Director, Clinical Operations
  Georgi Irvine, Commander (Ret), Nurse Corps, US Navy, Head, Medical and Dental Staff Services
- Drug Enforcement Administration, Office of Diversion Control
  Patricia Good, Chief, Liaison and Policy Section
  Sally Haskell, Liaison and Policy Section

- Educational Commission for Foreign Medical Graduates
  Stephen S. Seeling, JD, Vice President for Operations
  Liz Ingraham, Manager, Publications and Special Projects
- Federation of Medical Licensing Authorities of Canada
  Sylvia Smith, Executive Secretary
- Federation of State Medical Boards of the United States
  Patricia Beatty, Assistant Vice President
- Joint Commission on Accreditation of Healthcare Organizations
  Dennis O'Leary, MD, President
- National Board of Medical Examiners and United States Medical Licensing Examination Secretariat
  Kenneth E. Cotton
- National Association Medical Staff Services
  Becky Nichols, CEO
- National Committee for Quality Assurance
  Cary Sennett, MD, PhD, Executive Vice President
- National Practitioner Data Bank
  Robert Oshel, MD

The editors would also like to acknowledge the contributions of the following AMA staff:

- Physician Data and Internet Services
  Monica Quiroz and Julie Bain
- AMA Press
  Suzanne Fraker, Amy Roberts, Anne Serrano, Boon Ai Tan, and Ronnie Summers
- Medical Education Products
  Enza Messineo and Dorothy Grant
- Continuing Physician Professional Development
  Tina Blair and Charles Willis, MBA
- Healthcare Education Products and Standards
  R. Mark Evans, PhD
- Project USA
  John Naughton

Fred Donini-Lenhoff, Editor

Barbara S. Schneidman, MD, MPH, Vice President, Medical Education

Contents

List of Tables and Appendixes

Section I.

Licensure Policies and Regulations of State Medical Boards

·

State Medical Board Standards for Administration of the United States Medical Licensing Examination Steps 1 and 2

In 1990, the Federation of State Medical Boards (FSMB) and the National Board of Medical Examiners (NBME) established the United States Medical Licensing Examination (USMLE), a single examination for assessment of US and international medical school students or graduates seeking initial licensure by US licensing jurisdictions. The USMLE replaced the Federation Licensing Examination (FLEX) and the certification examination of the NBME, as well as the Foreign Medical Graduate Examination in the Medical Sciences (FMGEMS), which was formerly used by the Educational Commission for Foreign Medical Graduates (ECFMG) for certification purposes.

The USMLE is a single examination program with three steps. Each step is complementary to the others; no step can stand alone in the assessment of readiness for medical licensure. Each USMLE step is composed of multiple-choice questions, requires 2 days of testing, and is administered semiannually. Additional information on the USMLE appears on p. 62.

The majority of medical licensing authorities do not place any limits on the number of times a candidate for licensure may take USMLE Steps 1 or 2 or on the amount of time needed to complete both steps.

Additional Notes for Specific Licensing Jurisdictions

Texas—*Note A:* Applicants for licensure must pass each part of the USMLE within three attempts, but an applicant who has passed all but one part within three attempts may take the remaining part of the examination one additional time.

Notwithstanding the above, an applicant is considered to have satisfied the requirements if the applicant 1) passed all but one part of a board-approved examination within three attempts and passed the remaining part within five attempts; 2) is specialty board certified by an ABMS or AOA specialty board; and 3) completed an additional 2 years of board-approved GME in Texas.

Note B: An extension of the 7-year period for completing all three steps of the USMLE will be allowed for applicants who pursue a simultaneous MD/PhD or DO/PhD program. This extension will not exceed the second anniversary of the date the MD or DO degree was awarded.

State Medical Board Standards for Administration of the United States Medical Licensing Examination Step 3

(See the first two paragraphs on page 2 for general information on the USMLE.)

Many states require US or Canadian medical school graduates to have from 6 months to 1 year of accredited US or Canadian graduate medical education (GME) to take USMLE Step 3. Graduates of foreign medical schools are generally required to have completed more GME (as much as 3 years in several states). A number of states do not require completion of GME to take Step 3 or require only that a physician taking the examination be enrolled in a GME program.

Nearly all medical licensing authorities require completion of Steps 1, 2, and 3 within a 7-year period (exceptions are Rhode Island, which requires completion within 6 years; California and Kansas, which allow 10 years; and Idaho, Louisiana, Michigan, and New York, which do not impose a time limit). This 7-year period begins when the medical student or graduate first passes Step 1 or Step 2. Many licensing authorities also limit the number of attempts allowed to pass each step.

Additional Notes for Specific Licensing Jurisdictions

Florida—An extension of the 7-year period for completing all three steps of the USMLE will be allowed for applicants who pursue a simultaneous MD/PhD or DO/PhD program. This extension will not exceed the second anniversary of the date the MD or DO degree was awarded.

Ohio—All 3 Steps must have been passed within a 7-year period, and the performance achieved on each step must have been recognized by the USMLE as a recommended passing performance. A limited exception to this rule may be granted to an applicant who in conjunction with a medical degree is actively pursuing a doctoral degree in an institution or program accredited by the Liaison Committee on Medical Education and a regional university accrediting body. The applicant must be a student in good standing when enrolled in the institution or program, and the doctoral degree must be in a field of biological sciences tested in the Step 1 content. These fields include, but are not necessarily limited to, anatomy, biochemistry, physiology, microbiology, pharmacology, genetics, neuroscience, and molecular biology. Fields not excepted include, but are not necessarily limited to, business, economics, ethics, history and other fields not directly related to biological science. A limited exception to this rule may also be granted to an applicant who suffered from a significant health condition which by its severity would necessarily cause a delay to the applicant's medical study. Regardless, all three steps must have been passed within a 10-year period.

Texas—Note A: Applicants for licensure must pass each part of the USMLE within three attempts, but an applicant who has passed all but one part within three attempts may take the remaining part of the examination one additional time.

Notwithstanding the above, an applicant is considered to have satisfied the requirements if the applicant 1) passed all but one part of a board-approved examination within three attempts and passed the remaining part within five attempts; 2) is specialty board certified by an ABMS or AOA specialty board; and 3) completed an additional 2 years of board-approved GME in Texas.

Note B: An extension of the 7-year period for completing all three steps of the USMLE will be allowed for applicants who pursue a simultaneous MD/PhD or DO/PhD program. This extension will not exceed the second anniversary of the date the MD or DO degree was awarded.

Virgin Islands—The USMLE is not administered; SPEX is used to evaluate physicians' knowledge.

Washington—Individuals completing a dual profession program, in which the applicant has met the required 1 year of GME outside the 7 years from passing the first examination, are allowed an additional 3 years for the three attempts following completion of GME.

Table 1
State Medical Board Standards for Administration of the US Medical Licensing Examination Steps 1 and 2

	Number of Times Candidates for Licensure May Take USMLE Step 1	Number of Times Candidates for Licensure May Take USMLE Step 2	Amount of Time Within Which Steps 1 and 2 of USMLE Must Be Passed
Alabama	No limit	No limit	No limit
Alaska	1	1	7 yrs
Arizona	No limit	No limit	No limit
Arkansas	6	6	7 yrs
California	No limit	No limit	10 yrs
Colorado	No limit	No limit	No limit
Connecticut	No limit	No limit	No limit
Delaware	No limit	No limit	No limit
DC	No limit	No limit	No limit
Florida	No limit	No limit	No limit
Georgia	No limit	No limit	No limit
Guam	Not applicable	Not applicable	Not applicable
Hawaii	No limit	No limit	No limit
Idaho	2	2	No limit
Illinois	5	5	7 yrs
Indiana	No limit	No limit	No limit
Iowa	6	6	No limit
Kansas	No limit	No limit	No limit
Kentucky	No limit	No limit	No limit
Louisiana	No limit	4	No limit
Maine	No limit	No limit	No limit
Maryland	No limit	No limit	No limit
Massachusetts	No limit	No limit	No limit
Michigan	No limit	No limit	No limit
Minnesota	3	3	7 yrs
Mississippi	No limit	No limit	No limit
Missouri	3	3	No limit
Montana	No limit	No limit	No limit
Nebraska	4	4	No limit
Nevada	No limit	No limit	7 yrs
New Hampshire	3	3	7 yrs (all 3 steps)
New Jersey	No limit	No limit	7 yrs
New Mexico	6	6	7 yrs (all 3 steps)
New York	No limit	No limit	No limit
North Carolina	No limit	No limit	7 yrs
North Dakota	4	4	7 yrs

Table 1 (continued)
State Medical Board Standards for Administration of the US Medical Licensing Examination Steps 1 and 2

	Number of Times Candidates for Licensure May Take USMLE Step 1	Number of Times Candidates for Licensure May Take USMLE Step 2	Amount of Time Within Which Steps 1 and 2 of USMLE Must Be Passed
Ohio	No limit	No limit	7 yrs
Oklahoma	3	3	No limit
Oregon	No limit	No limit	No limit
Pennsylvania	No limit	No limit	No limit
Puerto Rico	No limit	No limit	7 yrs
Rhode Island	No limit	No limit	7 yrs
South Carolina	4	4	7 yrs
South Dakota	3	3	No limit
Tennessee	No limit	No limit	No limit
Texas	3	3 (see Note A)	No limit (see Note B)
Utah	3	3	7 yrs
Vermont	No limit	No limit	7 yrs
Virgin Islands	Not applicable	Not applicable	Not applicable
Virginia	No limit	No limit	No limit
Washington	No limit	No limit	No limit
West Virginia	No limit	No limit	7 yrs
Wisconsin	3	3	3 yrs
Wyoming	No limit	No limit	No limit

Table 2
State Medical Board Standards for Administration of the US Medical Licensing Examination Step 3

	Amount of Accredited US or Canadian Graduate Medical Education Required to Take USMLE Step 3		Number of Times Candidates for Licensure May Take USMLE Step 3	Amount of Time Within Which All Steps of USMLE Must Be Passed
	Graduates of US/Canadian Medical Schools	Graduates of Foreign Medical Schools		
Alabama	10 mos	2 yrs, 10 months	4	7 yrs
Alaska	1 yr	1 yr	1	7 yrs
Arizona	6 mos	6 mos	No limit	7 yrs
Arkansas	1 yr	1 yr	6	7 yrs
California	None	None	No limit	10 yrs
Colorado	1 yr	1 yr	No limit	7 yrs
Connecticut	None	None	No limit	7 yrs
Delaware	1 yr	1 yr	3	7 yrs
DC	1 yr	3 yrs	No limit	7 yrs
Florida	Not applicable	Not applicable	5	7 yrs
Georgia	1 yr	1-3 yrs	3	7 yrs
Guam	Not applicable	Not applicable	Not applicable	Not applicable
Hawaii	None (must be enrolled in first yr of GME prgm)	None (must be enrolled in second year of GME prgm)	No limit	7 yrs
Idaho	9 mos	2 yrs, 9 mos	2 (after 2 failed attempts, remedial training required)	No limit
Illinois	1 yr	1 yr	5	7 yrs
Indiana	6 mos	2 yrs (if passed ECFMG exam pre-7/84, 3 yrs GME required)	3	7 yrs
Iowa	7 mos	7 mos	3	7 yrs
Kansas	1 yr	2 yrs	3 (after 3 failed attempts, further education, training, or experience required to repeat exam)	10 yrs
Kentucky	1 yr	1 yr	No limit	7 yrs
Louisiana	None	None	4	No limit
Maine	1 yr	1 yr (plus ECFMG certificate)	3	7 yrs
Maryland	None	None	No limit	7 yrs (extended to 10 yrs for those in MD/PhD or similar programs)
Massachusetts	1 yr	1 yr	6	7 yrs
Michigan	6 mos	6 mos	No limit (after 5 yrs, further GME in a board-approved program in the state required to repeat exam)	No limit
Minnesota	None (but must be enrolled in GME prgm)	None (but must be enrolled in GME prgm)	3	7 yrs
Mississippi	1 yr	3 yrs	3	7 yrs
Missouri	1 yr	3 yrs	3	7 yrs
Montana	2 yrs (as of 10/1/01)	3 yrs	3	7 yrs
Nebraska	None	None	4	7 yrs
Nevada	1 yr	1 yr	No limit	7 yrs

Table 2 (continued)
State Medical Board Standards for Administration of the US Medical Licensing Examination Step 3

	Amount of Accredited US or Canadian Graduate Medical Education Required to Take USMLE Step 3		Number of Times Candidates for Licensure May Take USMLE	Amount of Time Within Which All Steps of USMLE Must Be Passed
	Graduates of US/Canadian Medical Schools	Graduates of Foreign Medical Schools		
New Hampshire	1 yr	1 yr	3 (after 3 failed attempts, further education, training, or experience required to repeat exam)	7 yrs (if not passed, must repeat entire sequence)
New Jersey	1 yr	1 yr	5 (after 5 failed attempts, further education, training, or experience required to repeat exam)	7 yrs (if not passed, must repeat entire sequence)
New Mexico	1 yr	1 yr	6 (within 7 yrs of first pass)	7 yrs
New York	None	None	No limit	No limit
North Carolina	1 yr	3 yrs	No limit	7 yrs
North Dakota	1 yr	1 yr	4	7 yrs
Ohio	1 yr	1 yr	No limit	7 yrs
Oklahoma	10 mos	10 mos	3 (after 3 failed attempts, on any part, specialty board certification required)	7 yrs
Oregon	None (but must be enrolled in GME prgm)	None (but must be enrolled in GME prgm)	No limit	7 yrs
Pennsylvania	None (but must be enrolled in GME prgm)	None (but must be enrolled in GME prgm)	No limit (after 3 failed attempts, further education required)	7 yrs
Puerto Rico	None	None	No limit	7 yrs
Rhode Island	1 yr	1 yr	4	6 yrs
South Carolina	1 yr	3 yrs	4	7 yrs
South Dakota	1 yr	1 yr	3	7 yrs
Tennessee	1 yr	1 yr	No limit	7 yrs
Texas	None	None	3 (see Note A)	7 yrs (see Note B)
Utah	None	none (must be ECFMG-certified)	3 (remedial training required after 3 failed attempts)	7 yrs
Vermont	1 yr	3 yrs	2	7 yrs
Virgin Islands	Not applicable	Not applicable	Not applicable	Not applicable
Virginia	1 yr (or enrolled in first year of program)	3 yrs (or enrolled in third year of program)	3	7 yrs (the Board may grant exceptions to this limit if good cause is shown)
Washington	1 yr (or enrolled in GME program)	1 yr (or enrolled in GME program)	3 (remedial training required after 3 failed attempts)	7 yrs (from time of first failure)
West Virginia	none	none	No limit	7 yrs
Wisconsin	1 yr	1 yr	3	7 yrs
Wyoming	1 yr	2 yrs	2	7 yrs

Abbreviations

USMLE—United States Medical Licensing Examination
ECFMG—Educational Commission for Foreign Medical Graduates
GME—graduate medical education

Note: *All information should be verified with the licensing board; medical licenses are granted to those physicians meeting all state requirements—at the discretion of the board.*

Endorsement Policies of State Boards for Physicians Holding an Initial License

Policies of medical/osteopathic licensing boards for endorsement of medical/osteopathic licensing examinations taken before and after the development of the Federation Licensing Examination (FLEX) vary from state to state. Each state board created its own licensing examination before FLEX, which may partially explain the sizable variation in endorsement policies from one state to another. Some boards will endorse scores on state licensing examinations in use prior to the development of FLEX, which may be endorsed in connection with a passing score on the Special Purpose Examination (SPEX). Endorsement of a certificate of the National Board of Medical Examiners (NBME) or of an examination refers to issuance of a license based on an acceptable score on the NBME or the state's board exam.

Endorsement relates to the issuance of licenses to physicians who hold licenses in other states or jurisdictions. Each state has strict endorsement requirements.

Forty-six state medical boards require some or all candidates for licensure endorsement to appear for an interview; eight boards require some or all candidates to appear for an oral examination.

Fourteen boards require that a license be endorsed within a certain period after examination (usually 10 years). In most of these 14 states, SPEX is required if the time limit is not met.

All medical boards will accept or consider for endorsement the national board certificate of the NBME or the United States Medical Licensing Examination (USMLE), except the Virgin Islands, which does not accept endorsements. The osteopathic boards in California, Michigan, Oklahoma, Pennsylvania, and West Virginia do not accept USMLE for licensure by endorsement.

Forty-three boards will endorse the Licentiate of the Medical Council of Canada (LMCC); 27 will endorse a state board examination (designated "SBE" in Table 3) from another jurisdiction, occasionally in combination with a certificate from an American Board of Medical Specialties (ABMS) specialty board; 7 will endorse an ABMS board certificate; and 26 will endorse the certificates of the National Board of Osteopathic Medical Examiners (NBOME). (Endorsement of these credentials is subject to any specific requirements in effect in that state.)

Additional Notes for Specific Licensing Jurisdictions

Colorado—LMCC is accepted or considered for endorsement for graduates of US or Canadian medical schools only.

Connecticut—Before June 1985: 75 on day 3 of FLEX to combine best scores (within 7 years); FWA truncated.

Delaware—A candidate who took FLEX more than three times before June 1985 will not be eligible for licensure by endorsement, unless the candidate completes 1 additional year of training acceptable to the board. In that case, SPEX will be required.

Idaho—FLEX scores obtained at different sittings cannot be combined. Applicants who fail to pass the FLEX or USMLE on two separate occasions will not be eligible to take the examination for at least 1 year, and before taking either examination again, they must show the board that they have successfully engaged in a course of study to improve their ability to engage in the practice of medicine.

Illinois—Applicant had to pass all three parts of the pre-1985 FLEX in the same state.

Louisiana—At Board discretion, candidates for licensure endorsement must appear.

SPEX may be waived if an applicant was certified or recertified by an ABMS board within 10 years of the application date.

Maryland—SPEX is required if active licensure was interrupted during the last 10 years and if physician has not passed a written licensure exam within the last 15 years and the ABMS certification exam within the last 10 years.

Minnesota—SPEX may be waived if the applicant was certified or recertified by an ABMS board within 10 years of the application date, or if the applicant is certified by a Canadian specialty board.

Mississippi—FLEX scores obtained at different sittings cannot be combined. An exemption may be granted to the weighted average of 75 on FLEX if the applicant has completed an approved GME program and is ABMS or AOA board certified.

LMCC is accepted or considered for endorsement for graduates of US or Canadian medical schools only.

SPEX may be waived if an applicant was certified or recertified by an ABMS board within 10 years of the application date.

Oregon—SPEX may be waived if an applicant was certified or recertified by an ABMS board within 10 years of the application date.

Texas—All candidates for licensure must appear, present original documents for inspection, and pass the Texas Medical Jurisprudence Examination.

Candidates who have not been examined for licensure in the preceding 10-year period prior to filing their application must pass the SPEX

-*or*- have passed a specialty certification/recertification examination or formal evaluation or an examination of continued demonstration of qualifications by an ABMS or Bureau of Osteopathic Specialist member board within the preceding 10 years

-*or*- have obtained, through extraordinary circumstances, unique training equal to the training required for specialty certification as determined by a committee of the board and approved by the board.

SPEX may be waived if an applicant was certified or recertified by an ABMS board within 10 years of the application date.

Table 3
Endorsement Policies of State Medical/Osteopathic Boards for Physicians Holding an Initial License

	Requirements for Endorsement of License Based on the Federation Licensing Examination (FLEX)			Requirements for Candidates' Appearance			Maximum Time for Licensure Endorsement After Examination		Credential Also Accepted or Considered for Endorsement (in addition to USMLE and NBME)
	Exceptions to 75 FWA on 3-part FLEX	Must Pass 3-Part (pre-1985) FLEX in One Sitting	Must Pass 2-Part (1985-93) FLEX in One Sitting	Candidates Who Must Appear...	...for Oral Exam	...for Interview	Time	Additional Requirements if Time Limit Not Met	
Alabama	None	No	No	Some			10 yrs	SPEX, ABMS	LMCC
Alaska	None	No	No	Some		X	None		LMCC, NBOME
Arizona	None	Yes	No	Some		Some	10 yrs	SPEX, ABMS	LMCC
Arizona DO	None	No	No	Some	X	X	7 yrs		NBOME, SBE (pre-FLEX)
Arkansas	None	Yes	No	IMGs		X	None		LMCC
California	None	Yes	No	None			10 yrs	SPEX	LMCC
California DO	None	No	No	All	X	X			NBOME
Colorado	None	Yes	No	None			None		LMCC
Connecticut	See note	No	No	None			None		LMCC, NBOME, SBE
Delaware	None	No	No	All		X	None	Training, SPEX	LMCC
DC	None	Yes	No	None			None		LMCC
Florida	None	Yes	No	Some		X	None		
Florida DO	NA	NA	NA	Some		X	None		NBOME, SBE
Georgia	None	Yes	No	Some		X	None		LMCC, NBOME
Guam	None	Yes	Yes	All		X	None		ABMS
Hawaii	None	No	No	None			None		
Hawaii DO	None	No	No	None			None		NBOME
Idaho	See note	Yes	No	Some	Some	Some	5 yrs	SPEX	LMCC, SBE, NBOME
Illinois	None	No	No	Some		X	None		LMCC, NBOME
Indiana	Split scores okay	No	No	Some		X	None		LMCC
Iowa	None	Yes	No	Some		X	None		LMCC, SBE
Kansas	No scrambled scores	Yes	No	Some		X	None		LMCC, SBE (pre-1972)
Kentucky	None	Yes	No	Some			None		
Louisiana	None	Yes	No	Some		X	10 yrs	SPEX	SBE
Maine	None	No	No	Some		X	None		LMCC, GMC, SBE
Maine DO	None	No	No	Some		X			NBOME
Maryland	None	Yes	No	None			15 yrs	SPEX	LMCC
Massachusetts	None	Yes	Yes	Some		X	None	Current evaluations	LMCC, NBOME
Michigan	None	Yes	No	None			None		LMCC, SBE
Michigan DO	NA	NA	NA	None					NBOME, SBE (pre-FLEX)
Minnesota	None	Yes (5 tries)	No (3 tries)	All		X	10 yrs	SPEX, ABMS	LMCC, NBOME, SBE
Mississippi	See note	Yes	No	All		X	10 yrs	SPEX, ABMS	LMCC, NBOME, SBE (pre-1973)
Missouri	None	Yes	No	Some		X	None		LMCC, NBOME
Montana	None	Yes	No	Some		X	None		LMCC

Table 3 (continued)
Endorsement Policies of State Medical/Osteopathic Boards for Physicians Holding an Initial License

	Requirements for Endorsement of License Based on the Federation Licensing Examination (FLEX)			Requirements for Candidates' Appearance			Maximum Time for Licensure Endorsement After Examination		Credential Also Accepted or Considered for Endorsement (in addition to USMLE and NBME)
	Exceptions to 75 FWA on 3-part FLEX	Must Pass 3-Part (pre-1985) FLEX in One Sitting	Must Pass 2-Part (1985-92) FLEX in One Sitting	Candidates Who Must Appear...	...for Oral Exam	...for Interview	Time	Additional Requirements if Time Limit Not Met	
Nebraska	None	Yes	No	None			None		LMCC, SBE
Nevada	None	No	No	Some		X	10 yrs	SPEX	ABMS (w/i 10 yrs of primary certification
Nevada DO	None	No	No	Some	Some	X			NBOME, SBE (pre-FLEX)
New Hampshire	None	No	No	None			None	May require exam, interview, proof of clinical competence, etc	LMCC, SBE
New Jersey	Pre-1/81: 74.5 FWA	No	No	Some		X	None		ABMS with SBE, LMCC plus ABMS and SBE
New Mexico	None	No	No	All		X	None		LMCC, SBE (pre-1974)
New Mexico DO	None	No	No	All		X			NBOME, SBE (pre-FLEX)
New York	None	No; 5-year period to pass all parts	No; 5-year period to pass all parts	None			None		LMCC (with a valid Canadian provincial license), ABMS, foreign license
North Carolina	1980-85: Day 1=70, Days 2 and 3=75	Yes	No	All	Some	X	10 yrs	Training, SPEX, AMA PRA	SBE, ABMS
North Dakota	None	Yes	No	Some		X	None		SBE, LMCC, NBOME, COMLEX
Ohio	72 if taken during first 2 yrs of a state's administration and accepted as passing by state	Yes	No	None			None		LMCC (professional experience in US or abroad)
Oklahoma	None	Yes	No	Some		X	None		LMCC
Oklahoma DO	NA			Some		X			NBOME
Oregon	None	Yes	No	Some		Some	7 yrs	SPEX	LMCC, NBOME
Pennsylvania	None	Yes	No	None			None		LMCC
Pennsylvania DO	None	No	No	None					NBOME, SBE
Puerto Rico	None	Yes	Yes	None			None		
Rhode Island	None	No	No	Some		X	None		LMCC, NBOME
South Carolina	Pre-6/85: 75 FWA with no daily score below 70	Yes	No	All		X	10 yrs	SPEX	SBE with ABMS
South Dakota	None	Yes	Yes	Some		X	None		LMCC
Tennessee	None	Yes	Yes	Some		X	None		LMCC, ABMS
Tennessee DO	None	No	No	Some	X	X			NBOME
Texas	None	Yes	No	All		X	10 yrs	SPEX	LMCC, NBOME, COMLEX
Utah	None	No	No	Some		X	None		LMCC, SBE
Vermont	None	Yes	Yes	All		X	None		LMCC, ABMS
Vermont DO	None	No	No	None					NBOME, SBE (pre-FLEX)

Table 3 (continued)
Endorsement Policies of State Medical/Osteopathic Boards for Physicians Holding an Initial License

	Requirements for Endorsement of License Based on the Federation Licensing Examination (FLEX)			Requirements for Candidates' Appearance			Maximum Time for Licensure Endorsement After Examination		Credential Also Accepted or Considered for Endorsement (in addition to USMLE and NBME)
	Exceptions to 75 FWA on 3-part FLEX	Must Pass 3-Part (pre-1985) FLEX in One Sitting	Must Pass 2-Part (1985-92) FLEX in One Sitting	Candidates Who Must Appear...	...for Oral Exam	...for Interview	Time	Additional Requirements if Time Limit Not Met	
Virgin Islands	No reciprocity or endorsement; All licensure candidates must sit for complete SPEX exam.								
Virginia	None	No (unless taken before 6/76)	Yes	Some		X	None		LMCC, pre-1970=SBE, with ABMS
Washington	None	No	No	None			None		LMCC (post-1969)
Washington DO	None	No	No	None					NBOME, SBE (pre-FLEX)
West Virginia	None	Yes	No	All		X	None		LMCC, SBE
West Virginia DO	NA	NA	NA	All		X			NBOME, SBE (pre-FLEX)
Wisconsin	None	Yes	No	Some	X	X	None		LMCC (post-1978)
Wyoming	None	Yes	No	All	X	X	None		LMCC

Abbreviations

FWA—Federation Licensing Examination (FLEX) Weighted Average, which applied to the pre-1985 three-part FLEX and gave greater weight to parts 2 and 3; all states currently require a minimum passing score of 75 on each component of the post-1985 two-part FLEX.

ABMS—certification from a member board of the American Board of Medical Specialties

FLEX—Federation Licensing Examination

GMC—General Medical Council of England and Ireland

IMG—International medical graduate

LMCC—certification by the Licentiate of the Medical Council of Canada

NBME—certificate of the National Board of Medical Examiners

NBOME—certificate from the National Board of Osteopathic Medical Examiners

SBE—state board examination

SPEX—Special Purpose Examination

USMLE—United States Medical Licensing Examination

Note: *All information should be verified with the licensing board; licenses based on endorsement are granted to those physicians meeting all state requirements.*

Additional Requirements for Endorsement of Licenses Held by International Medical Graduates

In all states, international medical graduates (IMGs) seeking licensure by endorsement must meet the same requirements as US graduates (listed in Table 3), in addition to the requirements in Table 4.

All states except West Virginia require that IMGs seeking licensure endorsement hold a certificate from the Educational Commission for Foreign Medical Graduates (ECFMG). In lieu of holding that certificate, a candidate for licensure in North Dakota may have passed a certification examination of an American Board of Medical Specialties (ABMS) board or, in Wisconsin, the Foreign Medical Graduate Examination in the Medical Sciences (FMGEMS).

About half of the boards require IMG candidates to have graduated from a state-approved foreign medical school; some also require 3 years of US or Canadian GME. A majority of jurisdictions also may require an interview or oral examination prior to endorsement.

Additional Notes for Specific Licensing Jurisdictions

California—Four years' licensure required for IMGs, in addition to 2 years of ACGME-accredited training (or 1 year of ACGME-accredited training plus ABMS, or 1 year of ACGME-accredited training plus SPEX).

Connecticut—State-approved foreign medical school must have been listed with the World Health Organization in 1970 (or by individual review).

Florida—Rules on clinical clerkships for IMGs adopted by the Florida Board before October 1986 do not apply to any graduate who had already completed a clinical clerkship or who had begun a clinical clerkship, as long as the clerkship was completed within 3 years.

Illinois—Candidate must have completed a 6-year postsecondary course of study, comprising 2 academic years of liberal arts instruction, 2 academic years in basic sciences, and 2 academic years in clinical sciences, while enrolled in the medical school that confirmed the degree.

Iowa—Requirement for graduation from a state-approved medical school is waived if candidate passed the Special Purpose Examination (SPEX) or state science examination, or completed 3 years of GME in an ACGME-accredited residency program, or held a permanent license to practice without restrictions in a US jurisdiction for at least 5 years.

Maryland—In addition to 2 years of ACGME- or AOA-accredited GME, 1 year of GME required if candidate failed any part of an examination three or more times and did not pass before 10/92.

Michigan—Candidate must have completed specific basic science courses and clinical clerkships in hospitals approved by the state board.

Minnesota—SPEX is required if candidate took initial licensing exam more than 10 years ago, unless candidate is ABMS or Canadian medical specialty board certified.

North Dakota—The ECFMG certificate requirement is waived for holders of the Fifth Pathway and for graduates of medical schools in Canada, England, Scotland, Ireland, Australia, or New Zealand. The requirement may be waived, by unanimous vote of the Board, for holders of ABMS certification.

The requirement for 3 years of US/Canadian GME is waived if the candidate holds an ABMS board certificate or has passed SPEX and (a) has successfully completed 1 year of state-approved GME in the US or Canada (or 3 years of GME in the United Kingdom), (b) has other professional experience and training equivalent to GME years 2 and 3, and (c) meets all other licensing requirements.

Rhode Island—Candidate must have obtained supervised clinical training in the US as part of the medical school curriculum in a hospital affiliated with an LCME-accredited medical school or an ACGME-accredited residency.

Texas—All IMG candidates for licensure must appear for interview, present original documents for inspection, and pass the Texas Medical Jurisprudence Examination.

Table 4
Additional Requirements for Endorsement of Licenses Held by International Medical Graduates
IMGs must also meet all the requirements for endorsement listed in Table 3

State	Candidate Must Have ECFMG Certificate	Candidate Must Have Graduated From a State-approved Foreign Medical School	Candidate Must Appear for...		Notes
			Interview	Possible Interview	
Alabama	Yes	Yes			SPEX (if no ABMS or SBE within 10 years)
Alaska	Yes	No		Yes	
Arizona	Yes	No			SPEX if exam is over 10 yrs (and no current ABMS)
Arkansas	Yes	Yes	Yes		
California	Yes	No			
Colorado	Yes	Yes			
Connecticut	Yes	Yes			
Delaware	Yes	No	Yes		
DC	Yes	Yes			
Florida	Yes	No		Yes	
Georgia	Yes	Yes		Yes	
Guam	Yes	Yes		Yes	
Hawaii	Yes	No			
Idaho	Yes	Yes		Yes	Possible oral exam
Illinois	Yes	No		Yes	
Indiana	Yes	No		Yes	
Iowa	Yes	Yes		Yes	
Kansas	Yes	No		Yes	
Kentucky	Yes	Yes			
Louisiana	Yes	Yes	Yes		3 years of GME in US required
Maine	Yes	No		Yes	Foreign medical school must be listed with ECFMG
Maryland	Yes	No			2 yrs of ACGME- or AOA-accredited GME required
Massachusetts	Yes	No		Yes	
Michigan	Yes	No			
Minnesota	Yes	Yes	Yes		SPEX and 2 years of GME in US required
Mississippi	Yes	Yes	Yes		
Missouri	Yes	Yes			
Montana	Yes	Yes		Yes	3 years of GME in US required
Nebraska	Yes	No			
Nevada	Yes	No			3 years of GME in US/Canada required
New Hampshire	Yes	No			
New Jersey	Yes	No		Yes	ECFMG cert. not needed from Fifth Pathway holders
New Mexico	Yes	Yes	Yes		Orientation required
New York	Yes	No			
North Carolina	Yes	Yes	Yes		
North Dakota	Yes (or pass ABMS)	Yes		Yes	3 yrs GME in US/Canada required
Ohio	Yes	No		Yes	
Oklahoma	Yes	Yes			

Table 4 (continued)
Additional Requirements for Endorsement of Licenses Held by International Medical Graduates
IMGs must also meet all the requirements for endorsement listed in Table 3

State	Candidate Must Have ECFMG Certificate	Candidate Must Have Graduated From a State-approved Foreign Medical School	Candidate Must Appear for... Interview	Possible Interview	Notes
Oregon	Yes	Yes		Yes	Foreign medical school must be listed with ECFMG 3 years of GME in US required
Pennsylvania	Yes	No			Foreign medical school must be listed with ECFMG 3 years of GME in US required
Puerto Rico	Yes	Yes			
Rhode Island	Yes	Yes	Yes		3 years of GME in US required
South Carolina	Yes	No	Yes		3 years of GME in US/Canada required
South Dakota	Yes	Yes		Yes	
Tennessee	Yes	Yes		Yes	
Texas	Yes	No	Yes		3 years of GME in US required
Utah	Yes	No		Yes	
Vermont	Yes	Yes	Yes		3 years of GME in US required
Virginia	Yes	No		Yes	Licensure in another state can replace ECFMG cert.
Washington	Yes	No			
West Virginia	No	No	Yes		3 yrs of GME in US required (or 1 yr plus ABMS cert.)
Wisconsin	Yes (or FMGEMS)	No			Possible oral exam
Wyoming	Yes	Yes	Yes		Foreign medical school must be listed with ECFMG

Abbreviations

ABMS—American Board of Medical Specialties

ECFMG—Educational Commission for Foreign Medical Graduates

FMGEMS—Foreign Medical Graduate Examination in the Medical Sciences

IMG—international medical graduate

SBE—state board examination

SPEX—Special Purpose Examination

VQE—Visa Qualifying Examination

Note: *All information should be verified with the licensing board; licenses based on endorsement are granted to those physicians meeting all state requirements.*

Policies of State Medical/Osteopathic Boards About the Special Purpose Examination (SPEX)

The Special Purpose Examination (SPEX), a 1-day, computer-administered examination with approximately 420 multiple-choice questions, assesses knowledge required of all physicians, regardless of specialty. SPEX is used to assess physicians who have held a valid, unrestricted license in a US or Canadian jurisdiction who are:

a) required by the state medical board to demonstrate current medical knowledge,

b) seeking endorsement licensure some years beyond initial examination, or

c) seeking license reinstatement after a period of professional inactivity. Physicians holding a valid, unrestricted license may also apply for SPEX, independent of any request or approval from a medical licensing board.

For more information on SPEX, see p. 71.

Fifty-one jurisdictions use SPEX to assess current competence or if a candidate has not taken a written licensure exam or the American Board of Medical Specialties (ABMS) board certification examination within a specified number of years (usually 10). In 24 jurisdictions, SPEX scores are valid for an unlimited length of time. Forty-one jurisdictions will accept SPEX scores from other licensing jurisdictions.

Additional Notes for Specific Licensing Jurisdictions

California—Four years' licensure in another state is required for international medical graduates.

Florida—SPEX is offered only to candidates who have actively practiced medicine for at least 10 years after obtaining a valid license in a jurisdiction or a combination of jurisdictions in the United States or Canada and who meet Florida's licensure requirements.

Maryland—SPEX is required if active licensure was interrupted during the last 10 years and if a physician has not passed a written licensure examination within the last 15 years and an ABMS board certification examination within the last 10 years.

Minnesota—SPEX scores are valid for an unlimited time, within three attempts.

North Dakota—SPEX (or ABMS board certification) is required when candidate is being considered for the following exception: If candidate has not completed 3 years of GME but has met all other licensing requirements and has successfully completed 1 year of US or Canadian GME in a board-approved program, and if the board finds that candidate has other professional experience and training substantially equivalent to the second and third years of GME, then candidate may be eligible for licensure.

Texas—SPEX scores accepted from other licensing jurisdictions if candidate passed with a score of 75 or higher.

Vermont DO—SPEX or COMVEX (Comprehensive Osteopathic Medical Variable purpose Examination), or both, may be required to reinstate an expired license.

Table 5
Policies of State Medical/Osteopathic Boards About the Special Purpose Examination

	SPEX May Be Required...	...for the Following Reasons	...to Assess Current Competence	...if Written Licensure Exam or ABMS Certification Exam Has Not Been Taken Within	SPEX Scores Valid for	SPEX Scores Accepted from Other Licensing Jurisdictions
Alabama	Yes	By board order	X	10 years	10 years	Yes
Alaska	Yes	To restore a retired license	X		No limit	Optional
Arizona	Yes	By board order	X	10 years	10 years	Yes
Arizona DO	Yes	By board order		10 years	10 years	
Arkansas	Yes	By board order	X			Yes
California	Yes		X	10 years	10 years	Yes
California DO	No					
Colorado	Yes	By board order	X			Yes
Connecticut	Yes		X			Yes
Delaware	Yes		X		No limit	Yes
DC	Yes	By board order	X			No
Florida	Yes		X		4 years	Yes
Florida DO	No					
Georgia	Yes	By board order	X			Yes
Guam	Yes	By board order	X			Yes
Hawaii	Yes	If MD took a state licensing exam			No limit	Yes
Hawaii DO	No					
Idaho	Yes	By board order	X		No limit	Yes
Illinois	Yes	Restore license after disciplinary action; if not been practicing for several years	X			Yes
Indiana	Yes		X			Yes
Iowa	Yes	If not been practicing for several yrs	X		No limit	Yes
Kansas	Yes	By board order	X		No limit	Yes
Kentucky	Yes	By board order	X		No limit	No
Louisiana	Yes		X	10 years	10 years	Yes
Maine	Yes	If not been practicing for > 1 yr	X		No limit	No
Maine DO	Yes	If not been practicing for > 1 yr or by Board order	X		No limit	No
Maryland	Yes			15 years	No limit	Yes
Massachusetts	No					No
Michigan	Yes	For those with clinical academic license				No
Michigan DO	No					
Minnesota	Yes	Restore license after disciplinary action	X	10 years	No limit	Yes
Mississippi	Yes	Restore license after disciplinary action	X	10 years	10 years	Yes
Missouri	Yes	Restore license after disciplinary action	X		No limit	Yes
Montana	Yes	If not been practicing or inactive Montana license for last 2 yrs	X	2 years	No limit	Yes
Nebraska	Yes		X			Yes
Nevada	Yes			10 years	10 years	Yes
Nevada DO	Yes	By board order	X			Yes
New Hampshire	Yes	By board order				No

Table 5 (continued)
Policies of State Medical/Osteopathic Boards About the Special Purpose Examination

	SPEX May Be Required...	...for the Following Reasons	...to Assess Current Competence	...if Written Licensure Exam or ABMS Certification Exam Has Not Been Taken Within	SPEX Scores Valid for	SPEX Scores Accepted from Other Licensing Jurisdictions
New Jersey	No					No
New Mexico	Yes	Restore license after disciplinary action; if not been practicing for several years	X		No limit	Yes
New Mexico DO	Yes	Determined on individual basis				
New York	Yes	Determined on individual basis	X	(if state board exam taken before 1968)	No limit	Yes
North Carolina	Yes		X	10 years	10 years	Yes
North Dakota	Yes	(see note on previous page)	X		No limit	Yes
Ohio	Yes	If not been practicing for 2 yrs	X		No limit	Yes
Oklahoma	Yes		X			Yes
Oklahoma DO	No	(COMVEX is used instead of SPEX)	X			
Oregon	Yes	If not been practicing for 1 yr, or no training or ABMS cert. for 10 yrs	X	10 years (or if state board exam taken before 1968)	10 years	Yes
Pennsylvania	Yes		X			Yes
Pennsylvania DO	No					
Puerto Rico	No					Yes
Rhode Island	No					No
South Carolina	Yes	Restore license after disciplinary action; if not been practicing for 2 yrs	X	10 years	10 years	No
South Dakota	No					No
Tennessee	Yes	Restore license after disciplinary action; if license retired > 5 yrs	X		No limit	Yes
Tennessee DO	No					
Texas	Yes		X	10 years	10 years	Yes
Utah	Yes	If not been practicing for several yrs; restore license after discipline	X			Yes
Vermont	No					No
Vermont DO	Yes	Restore license if not been practicing for > 1 yr				
Virgin Islands	Yes	To obtain licensure	X		No limit	No
Virginia	Yes		X		No limit	No
Washington	Yes	Restore license after disciplinary action; if not been practicing for 4 yrs	X		No limit	Yes
Washington DO	Yes		X		No limit	
West Virginia	Yes		X		No limit	Yes
West Virginia DO	Yes		X			Yes
Wisconsin	Yes	Restore license after disciplinary action; if not been practicing for several years	X		No limit	No
Wyoming	Yes		X			Yes

Abbreviations

ABMS—American Board of Medical Specialties

SPEX—Special Purpose Examination

Note: All information should be verified with the licensing board; medical licenses are granted to those physicians meeting all state requirements—at the discretion of the board.

Policies of State Medical/Osteopathic Boards for Initial Medical Licensure of US Medical/Osteopathic School Graduates

All states require a written examination for initial licensure—generally, for MDs, the three-step United States Medical Licensing Examination (USMLE), which has replaced the Federation Licensing Examination (FLEX) and the national board examination of the National Board of Medical Examiners (NBME). Osteopathic physicians take the three-level Comprehensive Osteopathic Medical Licensing Examination (COMLEX-USA) of the National Board of Osteopathic Medical Examiners (NBOME).

All osteopathic physicians must complete at least 6 months of a 1-year AOA- or ACGME-accredited program to be eligible to take Level 3 of the Comprehensive Osteopathic Medical Licensing Examination (COMLEX).

More than half of the state medical boards require graduates of US medical schools to have completed 1 year of graduate medical education (GME) to take USMLE Step 3. Seventeen boards do not require completion of any GME to take USMLE Step 3 (although in some cases a candidate must be enrolled in a GME program).

All medical and osteopathic boards require completion of at least 1 year of GME before issuing a full, unrestricted license.

Table 6
Policies of State Medical/Osteopathic Boards for Initial Licensure of US Medical School Graduates

	Amount of Accredited US or Canadian Graduate Medical Education Required	
	...to Take USMLE Step 3 or COMLEX Level 3	...for Licensure
Alabama	10 mos	1 yr
Alaska	1 yr	2 yrs (1 yr if completed medical school before 1/95)
Arizona	6 mos	1 yr
Arizona DO	6 mos of a 1-yr AOA- or ACGME-accredited program	1 yr AOA- or ACGME-accredited GME
Arkansas	1 yr	1 yr
California	None	1 yr (including 4 mos general medicine)
California DO	6 mos of a 1-yr AOA- or ACGME-accredited program	1 yr AOA- or ACGME-accredited GME, including at least 4 mos general medicine (unless applicant completed 1 yr of GME before 7/1/90). Straight psychiatry, pathology, or anesthesiology residencies not accepted.
Colorado	None (must be enrolled in GME prgm)	1 yr
Connecticut	None	2 yrs
Delaware	1 yr	1 yr
DC	1 yr	1 yr
Florida	None	1 yr
Florida DO	6 mos of a 1-yr AOA- or ACGME-accredited program	1 yr AOA-approved rotating internship
Georgia	1 yr	1 yr
Guam	1 yr	1 yr
Hawaii	None (must be enrolled in 1st year of GME prgm)	1 yr
Hawaii DO	None	1 yr AOA- or ACGME-accredited GME
Idaho	9 mos	1 yr
Illinois	1 yr	Entered GME pre-1/88, 1 yr; entered GME post-1/88, 2 yrs
Indiana	6 mos	1 yr (plus 1 yr GME if candidate failed any part of an exam 3 or more times and did not pass before 10/92)
Iowa	7 mos	1 yr
Kansas	1 yr	1 yr
Kentucky	1 yr	2 yrs
Louisiana	None	1 yr
Maine	1 yr	2 yrs
Maine DO	6 mos of a 1-yr AOA- or ACGME-accredited program	1 yr AOA- or ACGME-accredited GME
Maryland	None	1 yr (plus 1 yr GME if candidate failed any part of an exam 3 or more times and did not pass before 10/92)
Massachusetts	1 yr	1 yr
Michigan	6 mos	2 yrs
Michigan DO	6 mos of a 1-yr AOA- or ACGME-accredited program	1 yr AOA-approved GME
Minnesota	None (must be enrolled in GME program)	1 yr
Mississippi	1 yr	1 yr
Missouri	1 yr	1 yr
Montana	2 yrs (as of 10/1/01)	2 yrs (as of 10/1/01)
Nebraska	None	1 yr
Nevada	1 yr	3 yrs
Nevada DO	6 mos of a 1-yr AOA- or ACGME-accredited program	3 yrs in AOA-approved or ACGME-accredited prgm (grads after 1995)

Table 6 (continued)
Policies of State Medical/Osteopathic Boards for Initial Licensure of US Medical School Graduates

	Amount of Accredited US or Canadian Graduate Medical Education Required	
	...to Take USMLE Step 3 or COMLEX Level 3	...for Licensure
New Hampshire	1 yr	2 yrs
New Jersey	1 yr	1 yr
New Mexico	1 yr (must apply for public service license)	2 yrs
New Mexico DO	6 mos of a 1-yr AOA- or ACGME-accredited program	1 yr
New York	None	1 yr
North Carolina	1 yr	1 yr
North Dakota	1 yr (if not enrolled in in-state GME program; if enrolled in in-state program, can take at any time)	1 yr
Ohio	1 yr	1 yr
Oklahoma	10 mos	1 yr
Oklahoma DO	6 mos of a 1-yr AOA- or ACGME-accredited program	1 yr AOA-approved rotating internship or equivalent
Oregon	None (must be enrolled in GME program)	1 yr
Pennsylvania	None (must be enrolled in GME program)	2 yrs (1 yr if GME in US before 7/87)
Pennsylvania DO	6 mos of a 1-yr AOA- or ACGME-accredited program	1 yr AOA-approved rotating internship
Puerto Rico	None	1 yr
Rhode Island	1 yr	2 yrs
South Carolina	1 yr	1 yr
South Dakota	1 yr	2 yrs (completion of residency)
Tennessee	1 yr	1 yr
Tennessee DO	6 mos of a 1-yr AOA- or ACGME-accredited program	1 yr AOA-approved or ACGME-accredited GME
Texas	None	1 yr
Utah	None	2 yrs
Vermont	1 yr	1 yr (Canadian GME accepted if program accredited by RCPSC or CFPC)
Vermont DO	6 mos of a 1-yr AOA- or ACGME-accredited program	1 yr AOA-approved rotating internship or 3 yrs AOA- or ACGME-accredited GME program
Virgin Islands	USMLE not offered	1 yr
Virginia	1 yr (or enrolled in 1st year of program)	1 yr
Washington	1 yr (or enrolled in GME program)	2 yrs (1 yr if completed medical school before 7/28/85)
Washington DO	6 mos of a 1-yr AOA- or ACGME-accredited program	1 yr AOA-approved or ACGME-accredited GME
West Virginia	None	1 yr
West Virginia DO	6 mos of a 1-yr AOA- or ACGME-accredited program	1 yr AOA-approved GME
Wisconsin	1 yr	1 yr
Wyoming	1 yr	1 yr

Abbreviations

USMLE—United States Medical Licensing Examination

COMLEX—Comprehensive Osteopathic Medical Licensing Examination

GME—graduate medical education

RCPSC—Royal College of Physicians and Surgeons of Canada

Note: All information should be verified with the licensing board; medical licenses are granted to those physicians meeting all state requirements—at the discretion of the board.

Policies for Initial Medical Licensure of Canadian Citizens Who Are Graduates of Accredited Canadian Medical Schools

When considering applications for licensure, all state medical boards consider Canadian citizens who have graduated from an accredited Canadian medical school on the same basis as graduates of accredited US medical schools.

Forty-five licensing boards endorse the Licentiate of the Medical Council of Canada (LMCC) as evidence of passing an acceptable licensing examination (applicants must also pass all other board requirements for licensure).

With the exception of Guam, all medical boards accept Canadian graduation medical education (GME) as equivalent to GME in a US program accredited by the Accreditation Council for Graduate Medical Education (ACGME). These rules do not uniformly apply to international medical graduates, who should refer to Table 8.

Table 7
Policies of State Medical Boards for Initial Licensure of Canadian Citizens Who Are Graduates of Accredited Canadian Medical Schools

	Licentiate of the Medical Council of Canada (LMCC) Approved for Licensure by Endorsement	Graduate Medical Education in Accredited Canadian Programs Accepted as Equivalent to ACGME-accredited GME in the US	Notes
Alabama	Yes	Yes	
Alaska	Yes	Yes	
Arizona	Yes	Yes	
Arkansas	Yes	Yes	
California	Yes	Yes	
Colorado	Yes	Yes	
Connecticut	Yes	Yes	
Delaware	Yes	Yes	
DC	Yes	Yes	
Florida	No	Yes	
Georgia	Yes	Yes	
Guam	No	No	
Hawaii	No	Yes	
Idaho	Yes	Yes	
Illinois	Yes	Yes	Candidates who did not receive LMCC after 4/70 must be board certified or must complete USMLE Step 3 or the Special Purpose Examination
Indiana	Yes	Yes	
Iowa	Yes	Yes	LMCC must be endorsed by provincial licensing board
Kansas	Yes	Yes	
Kentucky	Yes	Yes	
Louisiana	No	Yes	
Maine	Yes	Yes	
Maryland	Yes	Yes	
Massachusetts	Yes	Yes	
Michigan	No	Yes	
Minnesota	Yes	Yes	
Mississippi	Yes	Yes	
Missouri	Yes	Yes	Only if medical school graduate of Canadian medical school
Montana	Yes	Yes	
Nebraska	Yes	Yes	
Nevada	Yes	Yes	
New Hampshire	Yes	Yes	
New Jersey	No	Yes	LMCC considered *only* if applicant is licensed in US jurisdiction
New Mexico	Yes	Yes	
New York	Yes	Yes	LMCC considered *only* if applicant has valid provincial license
North Carolina	Yes	Yes	LMCC accepted at board discretion
North Dakota	Yes	Yes	
Ohio	Yes	Yes	1 yr graduate medical education or its equivalent required

Table 7 (continued)
Policies of State Medical Boards for Initial Licensure of Canadian Citizens Who Are Graduates of Accredited Canadian Medical Schools

	Licentiate of the Medical Council of Canada (LMCC) Approved for Licensure by Endorsement	Graduate Medical Education in Accredited Canadian Programs Accepted as Equivalent to ACGME-accredited GME in the US	Notes
Oklahoma	Yes	Yes	
Oregon	Yes	Yes	
Pennsylvania	Yes	Yes	Must have received LMCC after 5/70 and in English
Puerto Rico	No	Yes	LMCC considered *only* if applicant is licensed in US jurisdiction
Rhode Island	Yes	Yes	
South Carolina	No	Yes	
South Dakota	Yes	Yes	
Tennessee	Yes	Yes	
Texas	Yes	Yes	
Utah	Yes	Yes	
Vermont	Yes	Yes	
Virgin Islands	No	Yes	LMCC accepted at board discretion
Virginia	Yes	Yes	
Washington	Yes	Yes	Must have received LMCC after 12/69
West Virginia	Yes	Yes	
Wisconsin	Yes	Yes	Must have received LMCC after 12/77
Wyoming	Yes	Yes	

Policies of State Medical Boards for Initial Licensure of International Medical Graduates

All international medical graduates (IMGs) must hold a certificate from the Educational Commission for Foreign Medical Graduates (ECFMG) examination before taking Step 3 of the United States Medical Licensing Examination (USMLE). For IMGs seeking licensure, Oklahoma is the only state that does not require an ECFMG certificate. (For more information on the ECFMG certificate, see p. 78.)

Thirty-seven states will endorse for licensure the Licentiate of the Medical Council of Canada (LMCC) when held by an IMG.

Fifteen state boards allow IMGs to take USMLE Step 3 before they have had GME in a US or Canadian hospital. All states, however, require at least 1 year of GME for licensure, and 27 states require 3 years. Candidates are not awarded a license until they undertake the required GME in the United States and meet other board requirements (eg, an ECFMG certificate, personal interview, payment of fees).

Fifth Pathway

In 1971, the AMA established Fifth Pathway, a program for US citizens studying abroad at foreign medical schools. The program requires that participants have

1. Completed, in an accredited US college or university, undergraduate premedical work of a quality acceptable for matriculation in an accredited US medical school, evaluated by measures such as college grade point average and scores on the Medical College Admission Test;

2. Studied medicine in a foreign medical school located outside the US, including Puerto Rico, and Canada that is listed in the *International Medical Education Directory*, available on the ECFMG Web site at www.ecfmg.org and developed and maintained by the Foundation for Advancement of International Medical Education and Research (FAIMER[SM]), a nonprofit foundation of the ECFMG.

3. Completed all formal requirements of the foreign medical school except internship and/or social service. (Those who have completed all the requirements of the foreign medical school are not eligible.)

If the aforementioned criteria are met, the candidate may substitute the Fifth Pathway program for internship and/or social service in the foreign country. After receiving a Fifth Pathway certificate from an accredited US medical school, these US citizens are eligible to enter the first year of GME in the United States.

In 50 states, individuals who hold Fifth Pathway certificates (but not the ECFMG certificate) are eligible for licensure. Fifth Pathway certificate holders must pass Steps 1 and 2 of the USMLE before entering a GME program accredited by the Accreditation Council for Graduate Medical Education (ACGME).

Additional Notes for Specific Licensing Jurisdictions

Florida—ECFMG certificate required for licensure if candidate is not a graduate of a foreign medical school approved by the Florida Board of Medicine (none has yet been approved).

Maryland—In addition to 2 years of ACGME- or AOA-accredited GME required for licensure, 1 year of GME required if candidate failed any part of an examination three or more times and did not pass before 10/92.

Maine—GME taken in Canada or the British Isles (accredited by a national body deemed equivalent to ACGME) may be considered qualifying on an individual basis.

Mississippi—ABMS board certification required for candidates who completed the Fifth Pathway.

North Carolina—IMG candidates for licensure must pass North Carolina board examination (USMLE or Federation Licensing Examination [FLEX]).

North Dakota—Three years of US or Canadian GME is required for licensure; if a candidate has not completed 3 years of GME but has met all other licensing requirements and has completed 1 year of GME in the United States or Canada in a board-approved program, and if the board finds that the candidate has other professional experience and training substantially equivalent to the second and third years of GME, the candidate may be deemed eligible for licensure (upon passing SPEX or ABMS board certification).

Oklahoma—An ECFMG certificate is not required for IMGs seeking licensure.

Oregon—IMG candidates for licensure must have completed at least 3 years of progressive GME in not more than two specialties in not more than two US or Canadian hospitals accredited for such training.

Pennsylvania—Board will grant unrestricted license by endorsement to a candidate who does not meet standard requirements if applicant has achieved cumulative qualifications that are endorsed by the board as being equivalent to the standard license requirements.

South Carolina—ABMS board certification required for candidates who completed the Fifth Pathway.

Wyoming—Oral examination is required for IMGs.

Table 8
Policies of State Medical Boards for Initial Licensure of International Medical Graduates

	Accepts Physicians Who Complete a Fifth Pathway Program as Candidates for Licensure	Endorses Canadian Certificate (LMCC) Held by an IMG	Amount of Accredited US or Canadian Graduate Medical Education Required	
			...to Take USMLE Step 3	...for Licensure
Alabama	Yes	Yes	2 yrs, 10 mos	3 yrs
Alaska	Yes	Yes	1 yr	3 yrs
Arizona	Yes	Yes	6 mos	3 yrs
Arkansas	Yes	Yes	1 yr	1 yr
California	Yes	Yes	None	2 yrs (including 4 mos general med)
Colorado	Yes	Yes/No (case-by-case review)	None (must be enrolled in GME)	3 yrs
Connecticut	Yes	Yes	None	2 yrs
Delaware	Yes	No	1 yr	3 yrs
DC	Yes	Yes (oral exam may be required)	1 yr	1 yr
Florida	Yes	No	None	2 yrs
Georgia	Yes	Yes	1-3 yrs	3 yrs
Guam	No	No	1 yr	2 yrs (varies by specialty; Canadian GME not accepted)
Hawaii	Yes	No	None (but must be enrolled in 2nd year of GME program)	2 yrs
Idaho	Yes	No	2 yrs, 9 mos	3 yrs
Illinois	Yes	Yes	1 yr	1 yr (entered GME pre-1988); 2 yrs (entered GME post-1988)
Indiana	No	Yes	2 yrs	2 yrs
Iowa	Yes	Yes (with valid Canadian provincial license and fulfillment of all other licensure requirements)	7 mos	1 yr
Kansas	Yes	Yes	2 yrs	2 yrs
Kentucky	Yes	Yes	1 yr	2 yrs
Louisiana	Yes	No	None	3 yrs (Fifth Pathway may be counted as 1 yr of required GME)
Maine	Yes	Yes	1 yr (plus ECFMG certificate)	3 yrs
Maryland	Yes	Yes	None	2 yrs AOA- or ACGME-accredited GME (as of 10/1/2000)
Massachusetts	Yes	Yes	1 yr	2 yrs
Michigan	No	No	6 mos	2 yrs
Minnesota	Yes	Yes	None (must be enrolled in GME)	2 yrs
Mississippi	Yes	No	3 yrs	3 yrs (or 1 yr plus ABMS certification)
Missouri	Yes	No	3 yrs	3 yrs
Montana	Yes	No	3 yrs	3 yrs (or ABMS or AOA certification)
Nebraska	Yes	Yes	None	3 yrs
Nevada	Yes	Yes	1 yr	3 yrs
New Hampshire	Yes	Yes	1 yr	2 yrs
New Jersey	Yes	No	1 yr	3 yrs (1 yr if medical school completed before 7/1/85)
New Mexico	Yes	No	1 yr (must apply for public license)	2 yrs

Table 8 (continued)
Policies of State Medical Boards for Initial Licensure of International Medical Graduates

	Accepts Physicians Who Complete a Fifth Pathway Program as Candidates for Licensure	Endorses Canadian Certificate (LMCC) Held by an IMG	Amount of Accredited US or Canadian Graduate Medical Education Required	
			...to Take USMLE Step 3	...for Licensure
New York	Yes	Yes (with valid Canadian provincial license and fulfillment of all other licensure requirements)	None	3 yrs
North Carolina	Yes	No	3 yrs	3 yrs
North Dakota	Yes	Yes	1 yr (if enrolled in-state, no GME required)	3 yrs
Ohio	Yes	Yes	1 yr	2 yrs (be enrolled in 2nd yr)
Oklahoma	Yes	Yes	10 mos	2 yrs
Oregon	Yes	Yes	1 yr	3 yrs
Pennsylvania	Yes	Yes (if passed after 5/70 and in English)	None (must be enrolled in GME program)	3 yrs (1 yr if GME taken in US before 7/87)
Puerto Rico	Yes	Yes	None	1 yr
Rhode Island	Yes	Yes (with valid Canadian provincial license and fulfillment of all other licensure requirements)	1 yr	3 yrs
South Carolina	Yes	No	3 yrs	3 yrs (plus ABMS certification)
South Dakota	Yes	Yes	1 yr	2 yrs (1 yr if US GME taken before 7/87) and completion of residency
Tennessee	Yes	Yes	3 yrs	3 yrs
Texas	Yes	Yes	None	3 yrs
Utah	Yes	No	None	2 yrs
Vermont	No	No	1 yr	3 yrs (Canadian GME not accepted)
Virgin Islands	Yes	No	Not applicable	1 yr
Virginia	Yes	Yes	3 yrs (must be in 3rd yr)	3 yrs
Washington	Yes	Yes (if passed after 12/69)	1 yr (or enrollment in GME program)	2 yrs (1 yr if medical school completed before 7/28/85)
West Virginia	Yes	Yes	None	3 yrs (or 1 yr plus ABMS certification)
Wisconsin	Yes	Yes (if passed after 12/77)	1 yr	1 yr
Wyoming	Yes	Yes	2 yrs	2 yrs

Abbreviations

GME—graduate medical education

IMG—International medical graduate

LMCC—Licentiate of the Medical Council of Canada

USMLE—United States Medical Licensing Examination

Note: *All information should be verified with the licensing board; licenses are granted to those physicians meeting all state requirements—at the discretion of the board.*

Medical Student Clerkship Regulations of State Medical Boards

For purposes of this publication, a clerkship is defined as clinical education provided to medical students. Twenty states evaluate the quality of clinical clerkships in connection with an application for licensure. In most states, clerkships for US medical students must take place in hospitals affiliated with medical schools accredited by the Liaison Committee on Medical Education (LCME). Twelve states have additional and/or more specific bases for evaluation.

Sixteen boards regulate clerkships provided in their states to students of foreign medical schools (including US citizens studying medicine in foreign schools). Of these, Pennsylvania, Puerto Rico, and Texas forbid such clerkships. For purposes of licensure, 19 states accept only those clerkships completed in hospital departments with graduate medical education (GME) programs accredited by the Accreditation Council for Graduate Medical Education (ACGME). Six states have additional unspecified regulations.

Additional Notes for Specific Licensing Jurisdictions

California—Students of foreign medical schools may complete up to 18 of 72 required weeks in nonapproved clerkships outside of California.

Florida—Rules on clinical clerkships for international medical graduates adopted by the Florida Board before October 1986 do not apply to any graduate who had already completed a clinical clerkship or who had begun a clinical clerkship, as long as the clerkship was completed within 3 years.

An international medical school must be registered with the Florida Department of Education for its students to perform clinical clerkships in Florida.

Texas—Acceptance of clerkships in hospital departments with ACGME-accredited programs applies to those outside of Texas but within the US.

Table 9
Medical Student Clerkship Regulations of State Medical Boards

State	Evaluates the Quality of Clinical Clerkships in Connection with a Licensure Application	Regulation of Clerkships Provided to Students of Foreign Medical Schools			
		Regulates Clerkships Provided by Hospitals	Forbids Clerkships for Students of Foreign Med. Schools	Accepts Clerkships Only in Hospital Departments with ACGME-accredited Programs	Has Other Unspecified Regulations
Alabama	Yes			Yes	
Alaska					
Arizona					
Arkansas	Yes*	Yes		Yes	
California	Yes*	Yes		Yes	Yes
Colorado					
Connecticut	Yes*	Yes		Yes	
Delaware	Yes	Yes		Yes	
DC	Yes	Yes		Yes	
Florida	Yes	Yes		Yes	Yes
Georgia	Yes*	Yes		Yes	
Guam					
Hawaii					
Idaho					
Illinois					
Indiana					
Iowa					
Kansas					
Kentucky	Yes	Yes		Yes	
Louisiana					
Maine	Yes			Yes	
Maryland					
Massachusetts	Yes*	Yes		Yes	Yes
Michigan					
Minnesota					
Mississippi					
Missouri					
Montana					
Nebraska					
Nevada					
New Hampshire					
New Jersey	Yes*	Yes		Yes	Yes
New Mexico	*				
New York	Yes*	Yes		Yes	Yes
North Carolina	Yes*			Yes	
North Dakota					
Ohio					
Oklahoma				Yes	
Oregon	Yes	Yes		Yes	
Pennsylvania	Yes*	Yes	Yes	Yes	

Table 9 (continued)
Medical Student Clerkship Regulations of State Medical Boards

State	Evaluates the Quality of Clinical Clerkships in Connection with a Licensure Application	Regulation of Clerkships Provided to Students of Foreign Medical Schools			
		Adopted Regulations Governing Clerkships Provided by Hospitals	Forbids Clerkships for Students of Foreign Med. Schools	Accepts Clerkships Only in Hospital Departments with ACGME-accredited Programs	Has Other Unspecified Regulations
Puerto Rico	Yes	Yes	Yes		
Rhode Island	Yes				
South Carolina					
South Dakota					
Tennessee					
Texas	Yes*	Yes	Yes	Yes	Yes
Utah					
Vermont					
Virgin Islands					
Virginia	Yes*	Yes		Yes	
Washington					
West Virginia					
Wisconsin					
Wyoming					
Total	**20**	**16**	**3**	**19**	**6**

In many cases, clerkships must take place in hospitals affiliated with Liaison Committee for Medical Education (LCME)-accredited medical schools or Accreditation Council for Graduate Medical Education (ACGME)-accredited residency programs. States requiring additional and/or more specific criteria for evaluation are asterisked (*).

Note: All information should be verified with the licensing board; medical licenses are granted to those physicians meeting all state requirements—at the discretion of the board.

Additional Graduate Medical Education and Specialty Certificate Policies of State Medical Boards

A number of state medical boards have additional graduate medical education (GME) and specialty certificate policies for international medical graduates (IMGs). Sixteen states have requirements for appointment to GME programs other than requiring an Educational Commission for Foreign Medical Graduates (ECFMG) certificate or a limited license.

Four boards—Connecticut, Maine, Nebraska, and Oklahoma—indicated that GME completed in foreign countries other than Canada may be considered for credit toward a license. Specialty certificates of foreign boards, such as the Royal College of Physicians in the United Kingdom, are accepted for credit toward a license in nine states.

Thirty-seven medical boards accept GME accredited by the Accreditation Council for Graduate Medical Education (ACGME) for licensure of osteopathic medical graduates.

Additional Notes for Specific Licensing Jurisdictions

Maine—May accept GME completed in England, Scotland, and Ireland for credit toward a license, if accepted by specialty board as meeting board eligibility in the United States and notified via certified letter.

Pennsylvania—IMGs seeking appointment to a GME program need a passing score on United States Medical Licensing Examination (USMLE) Steps 1 and 2 (or National Board of Medical Examiners [NBME] Parts I and II or Federation Licensing Examination [FLEX] Component 1) for graduate year 2 medical education; for graduate year 3 and above, all parts of USMLE (or NBME or FLEX) are required.

Table 10
Additional Graduate Medical Education and Specialty Certificate Policies of State Medical Boards

State	Has State Board Requirements for Appointment to GME Program Other Than ECFMG certificate or Limited License	May Accept GME Completed in Foreign Countries Other Than Canada for Credit Toward a License	May Accept Specialty Certificates of Foreign Boards (eg, Royal College of Physicians of the United Kingdom) for Credit Toward a License	Osteopathic Medical Graduates	
				ACGME-Accredited GME Accepted	State Osteopathic Board Handles Licensure
Alabama				Yes	
Alaska	Yes (residency permit required)				
Arizona	Yes (residency permit required)				Yes
Arkansas				Yes	
California	Yes				Yes
Colorado				Yes	
Connecticut	Yes (residency intern permit required)	Yes	Yes	Yes	
Delaware			Yes (case-by-case basis)	Yes	
DC				Yes	
Florida					Yes
Georgia					
Guam					
Hawaii					
Idaho				Yes	
Illinois				Yes	
Indiana				Yes	
Iowa	Yes (may require interview/exam)			Yes	
Kansas	Yes (residency intern permit required, and unapproved school must have been in existence at least 15 yrs)			Yes	
Kentucky	Yes			Yes	
Louisiana	Yes (passage of FLEX/NBME/USMLE)			Yes	
Maine		Yes	Yes	Yes	Yes
Maryland				Yes	
Massachusetts				Yes	
Michigan	Yes (certification of medical education)				Yes
Minnesota	Yes (residency intern permit required)			Yes	
Mississippi				Yes	
Missouri				Yes	
Montana				Yes	
Nebraska		Yes		Yes	
Nevada	Yes				Yes
New Hampshire				Yes	
New Jersey	Yes (residency intern permit required)			Yes	
New Mexico	Yes (residency intern permit required)				Yes
New York			Yes	Yes	
North Carolina				Yes	
North Dakota				Yes	
Ohio				Yes	

Table 10 (continued)
Additional Graduate Medical Education and Specialty Certificate Policies of State Medical Boards

	Has State Board Requirements for Appointment to GME Program Other Than ECFMG Certification or Limited License	May Accept GME Completed in Foreign Countries Other Than Canada for Credit Toward a License	May Accept Specialty Certificates of Foreign Boards (eg, Royal College of Physicians of the United Kingdom) for Credit Toward a License	Osteopathic Medical Graduates	
				ACGME-Accredited GME Accepted	State Osteopathic Board Handles Licensure
Oklahoma		Yes			Yes
Oregon				Yes	
Pennsylvania	Yes		Yes		Yes
Puerto Rico					
Rhode Island			Yes; may accept certificates of boards in England, Scotland, and Ireland	Yes	
South Carolina				Yes	
South Dakota				Yes	
Tennessee			Yes; specialty board must be AMA-recognized		Yes
Texas	Yes (physician-in-training permit required)			Yes	
Utah			Yes	Yes	Yes
Vermont	Yes		Yes; specialty board must be recognized by ABMS, RCPSC, or CFPC		Yes
Virgin Islands				Yes	
Virginia				Yes	
Washington					Yes
West Virginia					Yes
Wisconsin				Yes	
Wyoming				Yes	
Total	**16**	**4**	**9**	**37**	**14**

Abbreviations

ACGME—Accreditation Council for Graduate Medical Education

ECFMG—Educational Commission for Foreign Medical Graduates

FLEX—Federation Licensing Examination

GME—graduate medical education

NBME—certificate of the National Board of Medical Examiners

USMLE—United States Medical Licensing Examination

Note: All information should be verified with the licensing board; medical licenses are granted to those physicians meeting all state requirements—at the discretion of the board.

Accredited Subspecialties and Nonaccredited Fellowships That Satisfy GME Requirements for Licensure

Both the AMA and the Accreditation Council for Graduate Medical Education (ACGME) define a residency as graduate medical education (GME) that takes place in any of the medical specialties with ACGME Program Requirements (eg, internal medicine, pediatrics, surgery). Beginning in 2000, the ACGME has used the term "fellowship" to denote GME in ACGME-accredited subspecialty programs (eg, cardiovascular disease, vascular surgery, rheumatology) that is beyond the requirements for eligibility for first board certification in the discipline.

All state medical boards accept residency education in specialty programs accredited by the ACGME as satisfying their GME requirements for licensure. Forty-nine jurisdictions—all except Arkansas, Guam, Montana, Pennsylvania, and Puerto Rico—accept residency education in subspecialty programs accredited by ACGME as satisfying their GME requirements for licensure.

Six boards accept clinical fellowships not accredited by ACGME, and four boards—Hawaii, Missouri, New York, and North Carolina—accept research fellowships not accredited by ACGME to satisfy the GME requirement for licensure.

Table 11
Accredited Subspecialties and Nonaccredited Fellowships That Satisfy Graduate Medical Education Requirements for Licensure

	Accepts Subspecialty GME Accredited by ACGME	Accepts Clinical Fellowships *Not* Accredited by ACGME	Accepts Research Fellowships *Not* Accredited by ACGME
Alabama	Yes (if clinical)		
Alaska	Yes		
Arizona	Yes		
Arkansas			
California MD and DO	Yes		
Colorado	Yes		
Connecticut	Yes		
Delaware	Yes		
DC	Yes		
Florida	Yes		
Georgia	Yes		
Guam			
Hawaii	Yes	Yes	Yes
Idaho	Yes		
Illinois	Yes		
Indiana	Yes		
Iowa	Yes		
Kansas	Yes		
Kentucky	Yes		
Louisiana	Yes		
Maine	Yes		
Maryland	Yes		
Massachusetts	Yes		
Michigan	Yes		
Minnesota	Yes		
Mississippi	Yes		
Missouri	Yes	Yes	Yes
Montana			
Nebraska	Yes		
Nevada	Yes	Yes (with Board approval)	
New Hampshire	Yes		
New Jersey	Yes		
New Mexico	Yes		
New York	Yes	Yes	Yes
North Carolina	Yes	Yes	Yes
North Dakota	Yes		
Ohio	Yes		
Oklahoma	Yes		
Oregon	Yes		
Pennsylvania			
Puerto Rico			
Rhode Island	Yes		
South Carolina	Yes		
South Dakota	Yes		
Tennessee	Yes		

Table 11 (continued)
Accredited Subspecialties and Nonaccredited Fellowships That Satisfy Graduate Medical Education Requirements for Licensure

	Accepts Subspecialty GME Accredited by ACGME	Accepts Clinical Fellowships *Not* Accredited by ACGME	Accepts Research Fellowships *Not* Accredited by ACGME
Texas	Yes	Yes (if in Texas and Board-approved)	
Utah	Yes		
Vermont	Yes		
Virgin Islands	Yes		
Virginia	Yes		
Washington	Yes		
West Virginia	Yes		
Wisconsin	Yes		
Wyoming	Yes		
Total	**49**	**6**	**4**

Abbreviations

ACGME—Accreditation Council for Graduate Medical Education
GME—graduate medical education

Note: *All information should be verified with licensing board; medical licenses are granted to those physicians meeting all state requirements—at the discretion of the board.*

Licensure Requirement Exemptions for Eminent Physicians and Medical School Faculty

Twelve boards license physicians through recognition of eminence in medical education or medical practice. Physicians appointed to a medical school faculty are excused from the graduate medical education (GME) requirement for limited licensure in 15 states and from the examination requirement for limited licensure or teaching certification in 14 states. These faculty appointees would, however, receive a limited license or similar credential.

Additional Notes for Specific Licensing Jurisdictions

Colorado—Distinguished foreign physicians are invited to serve on faculty; temporary licensure may not exceed 2 years.

Florida—Physicians appointed to a medical faculty are eligible for a special license, with which they may practice only at the designated facility/institution.

Georgia—Physicians appointed to a medical faculty are excused from the GME requirement for limited licensure for teaching only.

Iowa—Physicians appointed to a medical faculty are eligible for a special license, with which they may practice only at the designated facility/institution.

Louisiana—Physician licensed through recognition of eminence in medical education must be approved as a tenured professor/associate professor by a Louisiana medical school.

Montana—An international medical graduate (IMG) seeking a restricted license must have published in an English-language, peer-reviewed medical journal.

New Hampshire—Courtesy license for educational purposes is provided to eminent physicians under limited circumstances.

Ohio—Physicians appointed to a medical faculty are eligible for a visiting medical faculty certificate, with which they may practice only at the school or teaching hospitals affiliated with the school. This nonrenewable certificate is valid for 1 year or the duration of the appointment, whichever is shorter.

Texas—Physicians appointed as full medical school professors in a salaried full-time position may be designated Distinguished Professors and be excluded from the Special Purpose Examination (SPEX) if required under the 10-year rule.

Table 12
Licensure Requirement Exemptions for Eminent Physicians and Medical School Faculty

	License Physicians Through Recognition of Eminence in Medical Education or Practice	Physicians Appointed to a Medical Faculty Are Excused From...	
		...the Graduate Medical Education Requirement for Limited Licensure	...the Examination Requirement for Limited Licensure
Alabama			Yes
Alaska			
Arizona		Yes	
Arkansas			
California MD and DO	Yes	Yes	Yes
Colorado			
Connecticut		Yes	Yes
Delaware	Yes		
DC	Yes		
Florida		Yes	Yes
Georgia		Yes (see note)	Yes
Guam			
Hawaii			
Idaho			
Illinois			
Indiana	Yes		
Iowa	Yes	Yes	Yes
Kansas			
Kentucky			
Louisiana	Yes	Yes	Yes
Maine			
Maryland	Yes	Yes	Yes
Massachusetts			
Michigan			
Minnesota			
Mississippi			
Missouri	Yes		Yes
Montana	Yes		
Nebraska			
Nevada			
New Hampshire	Yes (see note)		
New Jersey			
New Mexico			
New York			
North Carolina	Yes	Yes	Yes
North Dakota			
Ohio		Yes	
Oklahoma			
Oregon			
Pennsylvania	Yes	Yes	
Puerto Rico			
Rhode Island		Yes	Yes
South Carolina			

Table 12 (continued)
Licensure Requirement Exemptions for Eminent Physicians and Medical School Faculty

	License Physicians Through Recognition of Eminence in Medical Education or Practice	Physicians Appointed to a Medical Faculty Are Excused From...	
		...the Graduate Medical Education Requirement for Limited Licensure	...the Examination Requirement for Limited Licensure
South Dakota			
Tennessee		Yes	Yes
Texas			
Utah			
Vermont		Yes	Yes
Virgin Islands			
Virginia			
Washington			
West Virginia		Yes	Yes
Wisconsin			
Wyoming			
Total	**12**	**15**	**14**

Note: *All information should be verified with the licensing board; medical licenses are granted to those physicians meeting all state requirements—at the discretion of the board.*

Medical/Osteopathic Licensure and Reregistration Fees and Intervals; CME Reporting Requirements

The National Board of Medical Examiners (NBME) administers United States Medical Licensing Examination (USMLE) Steps 1 and 2 to students and graduates of US and Canadian medical schools at test centers established by the NBME; application materials are usually available at these medical schools. The Educational Commission for Foreign Medical Graduates (ECFMG) administers USMLE Steps 1 and 2 to students and graduates of foreign medical schools; application materials are available only through the ECFMG.

Administration of USMLE Step 3 is the responsibility of the individual medical licensing jurisdictions. Step 3 application materials for physicians who have successfully completed Steps 1 and 2 are available from the medical licensing authorities or the Federation of State Medical Boards (FSMB), which administers the examination for 48 jurisdictions (exceptions are Alabama, Illinois, and Puerto Rico). (For more information on USMLE Step 3 in those states where it is administered by the FSMB, call 800 USMLE XM—800 876-5396). The current fee for USMLE Step 3 in the 48 jurisdictions in which the FSMB administers the exam is $590. Most jurisdictions also have additional processing, application, and administrative fees.

For osteopathic physicians, the National Board of Osteopathic Medical Examiners (NBOME) administers the Comprehensive Osteopathic Medical Licensing Examination (COMLEX-USA) at various sites throughout the US. The Level 3 examination fee is $495.

Fees for licensure by endorsement, *including processing, application, and administrative fees*, range from $1,105 in California to $20 in Pennsylvania; the average is $291.

The majority of boards require physicians licensed in the state to reregister (or renew) their licenses every 1 or 2 years; four jurisdictions—Illinois, Michigan, New Mexico, and Puerto Rico—have a 3-year reregistration interval. The reregistration fee ranges from $500 per year in several states to $15 per year in Indiana; the average reregistration fee is $133 per year. Many states offer reduced fees for reregistration of inactive licenses (see Table 16 for more information).

Completion and reporting of a specified number of hours of continuing medical education (CME) is required for reregistration in 52 jurisdictions.

Additional Notes for Specific Licensing Jurisdictions

Arizona—If less than 10 years has elapsed since candidate passed a written examination for licensure in another state, endorsement fee is $550 (rather than $450), to include required Special Purpose Examination (SPEX).

Late penalty fee of $350 is charged if licensure reregistration is not submitted by February 1 of each year. License automatically expires on May 1 if renewal and late penalty fee are not submitted.

California—Endorsement fee includes $442 processing fee, $63 fingerprinting fee, and $600 licensing fee. Resident physician applicants are charged a reduced fee of $300.

Illinois—Reregistration fee for nonresidents is $600. Penalty of $100 is charged if renewal is not submitted by July 31 in the year of renewal.

Table 13
Medical/Osteopathic Initial Licensure, Endorsement, and Reregistration Fees and Intervals; CME Reporting Requirements

State	Examination						Endorsement Fees	Licensure Reregistration			Notes
	USMLE Step 3 Fee	COMLEX Level 3 Fee	Other Application Fees	Total Cost	Administered by			Registration Interval	Regular Fee	CME Reporting Required	
					FSMB	NBOME					
Alabama	$ 590		$ 195	$785			$ 175	1 yr	$ 200	Yes	
Alaska	590		840	1430	Yes		250	2 yrs	590	Yes	$250: Application fee for licensure endorsement
Arizona	590		500	1090	Yes		500	2 yrs	450	Yes	
Arizona DO		$ 495	400	895		Yes		2 yrs	600	Yes	
Arkansas	590		400	990	Yes		400	1 yr	70	Yes	
California	590		505	1095	Yes		1105	2 yrs	600	Yes	
California DO		495	505	1000		Yes	456	2 yrs	400	Yes	
Colorado	590		425	1015	Yes		375	2 yrs	305		
Connecticut	590		450	1040	Yes		450	1 yr	450		
Delaware	590		25	615	Yes		235	2 yrs	142	Yes	
DC	590		220	810	Yes		180	2 yrs	120		
Florida	590		815	1405	Yes		503	2 yrs	355	Yes	
Florida DO		495	605	1100		Yes		2 yrs	405	Yes	
Georgia	590		400	990	Yes		400	2 yrs	150	Yes	
Guam	590		400	990	Yes		400	2 yrs	250	Yes	
Hawaii	590		290	880	Yes		290	2 yrs	240	Yes	
Hawaii DO		495	290	785		Yes	400	2 yrs	190		
Idaho	590		300	890	Yes		400	1 or 2 yrs	200		Reregistration $200/yr
Illinois	604		300	904			300	3 yrs	300	Yes	$300 reregistration in state; $600 out of state
Indiana	590		250	840	Yes		40	2 yrs	30		
Iowa	590		50	640	Yes		400	2 yrs	325	Yes	
Kansas	590		300	890	Yes		300	1 yr	200	Yes	
Kentucky	590		615	1205	Yes		250	1 yr	125	Yes	
Louisiana	590		0	590	Yes		232	1 yr	132		$50 fingerprint fee
Maine	590		350	940	Yes		350	2 yrs	400	Yes	
Maine DO		495	350	845		Yes	350	2 yrs	400	Yes	
Maryland	590		790	1380	Yes		790	2 yrs	436	Yes	Endorsement/initial license $890 for IMGs
Massachusetts	590		600	1190	Yes		600	2 yrs	400	Yes	
Michigan	500		140	640	Yes		140	3 yrs	285	Yes	
Michigan DO		495	140	635		Yes		3 yrs	285	Yes	
Minnesota	590		200	790	Yes		200	1 yr	192	Yes	
Mississippi	590		500	1090	Yes		500	1 yr	150	Yes	
Missouri	590		300	890	Yes		300	2 yrs	200	Yes	
Montana	590		325	915	Yes		325	1 yr	200		
Nebraska	590		201	791	Yes		201	2 yrs	102		
Nevada	590		600	1190	Yes		400	2 yrs	600	Yes	
Nevada DO		495	500	995		Yes	200	1 yr	300	Yes	
New Hampshire	590		250	840	Yes		250	1 yr	150	Yes	
New Jersey	590		225	815	Yes		225	2 yrs	340		

Table 13 (continued)
Medical/Osteopathic Initial Licensure, Endorsement, and Reregistration Fees and Intervals; CME Reporting Requirements

| State | Examination | | | | | | Endorsement Fees | Licensure Reregistration | | | Notes |
	USMLE Step 3 Fee	COMLEX Level 3 Fee	Other Application Fees	Total Cost	Administered by FSMB	Administered by NBOME		Registration Interval	Regular Fee	CME Reporting Required	
New Mexico	590		462	1052	Yes		350	3 yrs	310	Yes	
New Mexico DO		495	300	795		Yes	300	1 yr	100	Yes	
New York	590		735	1325	Yes		735	2 yrs	600		
North Carolina	590		250	840	Yes		250	1 yr	100	Yes	$20 late fee if reregistration 30 days after birthday.
North Dakota	590		200	790	Yes		200	1 yr	150	Yes	
Ohio	590		335	925	Yes		335	2 yrs	305	Yes	
Oklahoma	590		400	990	Yes		400	1 yr	150	Yes	
Oklahoma DO		495	0	495		Yes	400	1 yr	200	Yes	
Oregon	590		375	965	Yes		375	2 yrs	438		
Pennsylvania	590		35	625	Yes		20	2 yrs	360		Endorsement $80 for IMGs
Pennsylvania DO		495	30	525		Yes		2 yrs	140		
Puerto Rico	500		0	500			200	3 yrs	75	Yes	
Rhode Island	590		350	940	Yes		350	1 yr	200	Yes	
South Carolina	590		0	590	Yes		500	1 yr	90	Yes	
South Dakota	590		200	790	Yes		200	1 yr	50		
Tennessee	590		290	880	Yes		235	2 yrs	160		
Tennessee DO		495	285	780		Yes		2 yrs	170	Yes	
Texas	590		800	1390	Yes		800	1 yr	330	Yes	
Utah	590		180	770	Yes		180	2 yrs	100	Yes	
Vermont	590		350	840	Yes		400	2 yrs	350		
Vermont DO		495	300	795		Yes		2 yrs	350	Yes	
Virgin Islands	NA	NA	NA	NA			NA	1 yr	500	Yes	
Virginia	590		225	815	Yes		225	2 yrs	260	Yes	
Washington	590		300	890	Yes		300	2 yrs	450	Yes	Add $25 for initial license endorsement
Washington DO		495	650	1145		Yes	650	1 yr	475	Yes	
West Virginia	590		600	1190	Yes		300	2 yrs	300	Yes	
West Virginia DO		495	200	695		Yes	200	2 yrs	200	Yes	
Wisconsin	590		68	658	Yes		110	2 yrs	110	Yes	
Wyoming	590		350	940	Yes		350	1 yr	200		
Total/Average	**$590**	**$495**	**$285**	**$715**			**291**		**133**	**52**	

Abbreviations

CME—continuing medical education
FSMB—Federation of State Medical Boards
IMG—international medical graduate
USMLE—United States Medical Licensing Examination

Note: *All information should be verified with the licensing board; medical licenses are granted to those physicians meeting all state requirements—at the discretion of the board.*

Continuing Medical Education for Licensure Reregistration

Fifty-two boards require anywhere from 12 hours (Alabama) to 50 hours (several states) of continuing medical education (CME) per year for license reregistration. Some states also mandate CME content, such as HIV/AIDS, risk management, or medical ethics. In addition, many states also require that a certain percentage of CME be category 1, as measured, for example, through the American Medical Association Physician's Recognition Award.

Additional Notes for Specific Licensing Jurisdictions

California—All general internists and family physicians who have a patient population of which over 25% are 65 years of age or older shall complete at least 20% of all mandatory continuing education hours in a course on geriatric medicine or the care of older patients.

All physicians and surgeons shall complete a mandatory continuing education course in the subjects of pain management the treatment of terminally ill and dying patients (one-time requirement of 12 credit hours, to be completed by December 31, 2006). Physicians practicing in pathology or radiology specialty areas are exempt from this requirement.

Florida—Physicians may complete a 1-hour CME course on end-of-life and palliative health care in lieu of the required 1-hour CME course on HIV/AIDS, provided the physician completed the HIV/AIDS course in the immediately preceding biennium (2-year licensure term).

Physicians may complete a 1-hour CME course on end-of-life and palliative health care in lieu of the required 1-hour CME course on domestic violence, provided the physician completed the domestic violence course in the immediately preceding biennium (2-year licensure term).

Maryland—Partial CME credit is offered for ABMS certification, select peer review, serving as a intervenor or monitor on a physician rehabilitation committee or professional committee, and serving as a preceptor for resident physicians or medical students in LCME-accredited schools. For first license renewal, CME requirement is waived, but licensee must have completed an approved orientation program.

Table 14
State Medical/Osteopathic Board Regulations on Continuing Medical Education for Licensure Reregistration

State	Required Number of CME Hours per Year(s)		Average Hours per Year	AMA/AOA/AAFP/ACOG Category 1 Hours Required	Certificates Accepted as Equivalent*	State-mandated CME Content/ Additional Notes
Alabama	24	2 yrs	12	24	ACOG, AAFP	
Alaska	34	2 yrs	17	17	AMA PRA, ABMS, AOA, APA	
Arizona	40	2 yrs	20		ABMS, GME	40 hours within 2-year timeframe
Arizona DO	20	1 yr	20	20		20 hours Category 1-A only
Arkansas	20	1 yr	20	20	AMA PRA	
California	100	4 yrs	25	100	AMA PRA, AAFP, CMA, CAFP	Pain management/geriatric medicine (see note)
California DO	150	3 yrs	50	90	AMA PRA, AAFP, CMA, CAFP, AOA	60 hours Category 1-A or 1-B
Colorado	none					
Connecticut	none					
Delaware	40	2 yrs	20	40	AMA PRA, AOA	
DC	none					
Florida	40	2 yrs	20	40		HIV/AIDS, domestic violence, TB
Florida DO	40	2 yrs	20	20 (AOA)		HIV/AIDS, domestic violence, risk management, FL rules/laws, managed care
Georgia	40	2 yrs	20	40	AMA PRA, AOA, AAFP, ACOG, ACEP	
Guam	100	2 yrs	50	25		
Hawaii	40	2 yrs	20	40	AMA PRA	
Hawaii DO	none					
Idaho	none					
Illinois	150	3 yrs	50	60	AMA PRA, AOA	
Indiana	none					
Iowa	40	2 yrs	20	40		Child/dependent adult abuse
Kansas	50	1 yr	50	20	AMA PRA, ABMS, GME, AOA	
Kentucky	60	3 yrs	20	30	AMA PRA	HIV/AIDS; course must be approved by Kentucky Cabinet for Hlth Svcs
Louisiana	20	1 yr	20	20	AMA PRA	One-time Board Orientation course
Maine	100	2 yrs	50	40	AMA PRA, ABMS, AAFP	
Maine DO	100	2 yrs	50	40		
Maryland	50	2 yrs	25	50		(see note)
Massachusetts	100	2 yrs	50	40	AMA PRA, GME	Study board reqs; risk mgmt
Michigan	150	3 yrs	50	75		
Michigan DO	150	3 yrs	50	60		60 hours Category 1-A or 1-B
Minnesota	75	3 yrs	25	75	AMA PRA, AOA, MOCOMP	
Mississippi	40	2 yrs	20	40	ABMS, AOA, AAFP, ACOG	
Missouri	25	1 yr	25		AAFP	
Montana	none					
Nebraska	none					
Nevada	40	2 yrs	20	40		ethics (2 hrs), 20 hrs in specialty
Nevada DO	35	1 yr	35	35		
New Hampshire	150	3 yrs	50	60	AMA PRA, ABMS	Credits reported to NH Med Society

Table 14 (continued)
State Medical/Osteopathic Board Regulations on Continuing Medical Education for Licensure Reregistration

State	Required Number of CME Hours per Year(s)		Average Hours per Year	AMA/AOA/AAFP/ACOG Category 1 Hours Required	Certificates Accepted as Equivalent*	State-mandated CME Content/ Additional Notes
New Jersey	none					
New Mexico	75	3 yrs	25	75	AMA PRA, ABMS, AAFP, ACOG, USMLE	
New Mexico DO	75	3 yrs	25	75	AMA PRA, ABMS, AAFP, ACOG, USMLE	Active membership in AOA may replace 75 hours of CME
New York	none					infection control, child abuse
North Carolina	150	3 yrs	50	0		
North Dakota	20	1 yr	20	20	AMA PRA, AOA, AAFP, MOCOMP	
Ohio	100	2 yrs	50	40	AMA PRA	All CME must be certified by the OSMA or OOA
Oklahoma	150	3 yrs	50	60	AMA PRA, ABMS	
Oklahoma DO	16	1 yr	16	16		16 hrs of Category 1, 1 hr of which must be CME on prescribing controlled substances (every 2 yrs)
Oregon	none					
Pennsylvania	none					150 hrs of CME every 3 years required by state insurance agency
Pennsylvania DO	100	2 yrs	50	20		20 hrs of Category 1-A or 1-B
Puerto Rico	60	3 yrs	20	40		
Rhode Island	60	3 yrs	20	60		HIV universal precautions/ blood-borne pathogens
South Carolina	40	2 yrs	20	40	ABMS, AOA, ACOG equivalent	
South Dakota	none					
Tennessee	none					
Tennessee DO	50	2 yrs	25	50		
Texas	24	1 yr	24	12		Of 12 hrs category 1, at least 1 hr in ethics/prof. responsibility
Utah	40	2 yrs	20	40	AMA PRA	
Vermont	none					
Vermont DO	30	2 yrs	15			At least 12 of 30 hours must be osteopathic med education
Virgin Islands	40	1 yr	40	25		
Virginia	60	2 yrs	30	30	AMA PRA	Of category 1, 15 hrs must be interactive
Washington	200	4 yrs	50		AMA PRA, ABMS, AAFP, ACOG	
Washington DO	150	3 yrs	50	60		
West Virginia	50	2 yrs	25	50	AMA PRA, ABMS (partial)	2 hrs end-of-life pain management
West Virginia DO	32	2 yrs	16	16	Board-recognized equivalent	2 hrs end-of-life management
Wisconsin	30	2 yrs	15	30	AMA PRA	
Wyoming	none					

ABMS—certification or recertification by a member board of the American Board of Medical Specialties; **AMA PRA**—American Medical Association Physician's Recognition Award; **AOA**—American Osteopathic Association; **AAFP**—American Academy of Family Practice; **ACOG**—American College of Obstetricians and Gynecologists; **APA**—American Pediatric Association; **CMA**—California Medical Association; **CAFP**—California Academy of Family Physicians; **CME**—continuing medical education; **FLEX**—Federation Licensing Examination; **GME**—graduate medical education; **MOCOMP**—Royal College of Physicians and Surgeons of Canada; **OSMA**—Ohio State Medical Association; **USMLE**—United States Medical Licensing Association

Note: All information should be verified with the licensing board; medical licenses are granted to those physicians meeting all state requirements—at the discretion of the board.

Teaching and Resident Physician Licenses Issued by State Medical/Osteopathic Boards

Fifty-eight jurisdictions issue educational licenses, permits, certificates, or registration to resident physicians in graduate medical education (GME) programs, with fees ranging from zero to $225 per year. (The GME program director generally provides a list of residents and any other required information directly to the licensing jurisdiction.) In 31 of those jurisdictions, residents must obtain a new permit/license when changing residency programs within the state.

Medical boards in 10 states—Arizona, California, Indiana, Kentucky, Maine, Massachusetts, Mississippi, New Hampshire, New Mexico, and Oklahoma—require that prospective residents have passed United States Medical Licensing Examination (USMLE) Step 1 to receive a permit/license. California and Mississippi require passage of Steps 1 and 2.

Thirty-nine jurisdictions issue teaching (visiting professor) licenses, with fees ranging from zero to $400.

Additional Notes for Specific Licensing Jurisdictions

California—Renewable certificates of registration (awarded on an individual basis) for 1-5 years to physicians who do not immediately meet licensure requirements and who have been offered full-time teaching positions in California medical schools.

Permits (awarded on an individual basis) for maximum of 5 years to noncitizen physicians for postgraduate work in a California medical school.

IMGs must submit an application to determine that all core requirements have been met before they may begin training in California.

Biennially renewable faculty permit (awarded on an individual basis) issued to academically eminent physicians, for whom the medical school has assumed direct responsibility. The holder may practice medicine only within the sponsoring medical school and affiliated institutions.

Florida—A Medical Faculty Certificate is granted to MDs who are graduates of an accredited medical school or its equivalent and hold a valid current license to practice medicine in another US jurisdiction. Certificate authorizes practice only in conjunction with teaching duties at an accredited Florida medical school or in its main teaching hospitals. A 180-day permit; no more than three physicians per year per institution may hold this certificate; certificate can be granted to a physician only once in a given 5-year period.

Illinois—Limited temporary licenses (valid for 6 months) to persons in non-Illinois residency programs who are accepted for a specific period of time to perform a portion of that program at a clinical residency program in Illinois due to the lack of adequate facilities in their state.

Visiting Professor Permits for 1 year (renewable once) to persons receiving faculty appointments to teach in either a medical or osteopathic school.

Visiting Physician Permits for up to 180 days to persons receiving an invitation or appointment to study, demonstrate, or perform a specific medical, osteopathic, or chiropractic subject or technique in medical, osteopathic, or chiropractic schools; hospitals; or facilities operated pursuant to the Ambulatory Surgical Treatment Center Act.

Visiting Resident Permits issued for 180 days to persons who have been invited or appointed for a specific period of time to perform a portion of that clinical residency program under the supervision of an Illinois-licensed physician in an Illinois patient care clinic or facility affiliated with the out-of-state GME program.

Massachusetts—Limited registration for physicians enrolled in accredited residency programs and for physicians enrolled in fellowships at hospitals with accredited residency programs in the area of the applicant's specialty.

Temporary registration for physicians who hold a temporary faculty appointment at a Massachusetts medical school, are substituting temporarily for a fully licensed Massachusetts physician, or are enrolled in a CME course that requires Massachusetts licensure.

Physicians requesting temporary registration must be currently licensed in another state.

Mississippi—Institutional license to interns and IMG physicians providing health care in state institutions. Applicants are not required to meet all requirements for permanent unrestricted licensure.

Restricted temporary license to physicians enrolled in first year of graduate medical education at the University of Mississippi School of Medicine for practice limited to that school.

Addictionology Fellowship License to physicians admitted for treatment in a board-approved drug and/or alcohol addiction treatment program or to physicians enrolled in fellowship of addictionology of the Mississippi State Medical Association Impaired Professionals Program.

Oregon—Limited License for Visiting Professor (VP), Medical Faculty (MF), SPEX, Special, Postgraduate (PG), and Fellow, which may be valid up to 1 year. LL-VP and Fellow licenses may be renewed for 1 additional year, LL-MF for 3 additional years, LL-PG annually until training is completed.

LL-VP valid for a 1-year teaching position.

LL-MF valid for a full-time faculty position offered by dean of medical school.

Pennsylvania—Interim Limited License (up to 12 consecutive months) to physicians providing medical service other than at the training location of the licensee's accredited GME program.

Graduate License allows licensee to participate for a period of up to 12 consecutive months in GME within the complex of the hospital to which the licensee is assigned and any satellite facility or other training location used in the program.

Institutional License allows qualified person to teach and/or practice medicine for a period of time not to exceed 3 years in one of the Commonwealth's medical colleges, its affiliates, or community hospitals.

Temporary License allows licensee to teach medicine and surgery or participate in a medical procedure necessary for the well-being of a specified patient within the Commonwealth. Applicants for a temporary license must hold an unrestricted license in another state, territory, possession, or country.

Table 15
Teaching (Visiting Professor) and Resident Physician Licenses Issued by State Medical/Osteopathic Boards

	Residents and Prospective Residents			Teaching (Visiting Professor) Licenses	Notes
	Licenses, Permits, Certificates, & Registration	Must Obtain New Permit/License When Changing Residency Programs Within State	Prospective Residents Applying for License Must Have Passed USMLE Step 1		
Alabama				Yes	Limited license for residency education only.
Alaska	Yes				Residency permits for up to 18 mos. to physicians in accredited residency programs in the US
Arizona	Yes, $25/yr	Yes	Yes	Yes, $100	Education Training Permit, granted for 5 days. Teaching licenses, for practice within clinical training program only, granted to full-time faculty members at an accredited medical school or GME program.
Arizona DO	Yes			Yes, $300	Education Training Permit, granted for 5 days, $100.
Arkansas					
California	Yes		Yes	Yes	
California DO				Yes	
Colorado	Yes, $20	Yes		Yes, $100	Training license valid for duration of program; renews every 3 yrs
Connecticut	Yes, $0	Yes		Yes, $0	
Delaware	Yes, $0	Yes		Yes	Limited institutional license under supervision of licensed physician
DC					
Florida	Yes, $100	Yes		Yes	
Florida DO	Yes, $100	Yes		Yes, $400	Faculty certificate; unlicensed registration number (for residents)
Georgia				Yes	Teacher's license for faculty of approved Georgia medical schools.
Guam	Yes	Yes			
Hawaii	Yes, $75				
Hawaii DO	Yes				
Idaho	Yes, $10				
Illinois	Yes	Yes		Yes	
Indiana	Yes, $50	Yes	Yes	Yes, $50	Resident permit good for 1 yr, may be renewed annually. Visiting professor license granted to an institution for a specific physician to whom it has granted a visiting faculty appointment. Institution must certify the physician's qualifications; physician's practice limited to the institution for designated period not to exceed 1 yr.
Iowa	Yes, $75	Yes		Yes, $200	Resident physician license for training in approved hospital under supervision of licensed physician.
Kansas	Yes, $40			Yes, $25	
Kentucky	Yes, $75		Yes		Institutional Practice Limited License or Residency Training License to physicians beyond first year of GME while still in training.
Louisiana	Yes, $25	Yes		Yes	Intern registration for first 12 months of GME after completing medical school.
Maine	Yes, $50	Yes	Yes	Yes, $0	Educational permits for 1 year in a specific training program, renewable for 5 years.
Maine DO	Yes, $200	Yes		Yes, $0	Temp. educational permits for 1 yr in a specific training pgm only
Maryland	Yes			Yes, $300	Registration of med school grads in GME programs. Limited 1-year license for graduate teaching.
Massachusetts	Yes, $100	Yes	Yes	Yes, $250	
Michigan	Yes, $80	Yes		Yes, $80	Limited annual license (not to exceed 5 years) for GME, renewable each year.

Table 15 (continued)
Teaching (Visiting Professor) and Resident Physician Licenses Issued by State Medical/Osteopathic Boards

	Residents and Prospective Residents			Teaching (Visiting Professor) Licenses	Notes
	Licenses, Permits, Certificates, & Registration	Must Obtain New Permit/License When Changing Residency Programs Within State	Prospective Residents Applying for License Must Have Passed USMLE Step 1		
Michigan DO	Yes, $80				
Minnesota	Yes	Yes			
Mississippi	Yes, $50/$200		Yes (and Step 2)		
Missouri	Yes, $30	Yes		Yes	Temporary licenses issued to interns, residents, and fellows only.
Montana					
Nebraska	Yes, $25	Yes		Yes, $25	Temporary educational permits for residents and temporary visiting faculty permits for medical school faculty.
Nevada	Yes, $250	Yes			Limited 1-yr license to residents in a clinical program ($250 initial fee, $50 renewal)
Nevada DO	Yes, $50	Yes		Yes, $50	
New Hampshire	Yes, $150	Yes	Yes	Yes, $50	
New Jersey	Yes, $50	Yes			Residency training permit required for unlicensed residents in GY2+
New Mexico	Yes, $10		Yes	Yes, $100	
New Mexico DO	Yes, $25				
New York	Yes, $105				Requires limited permit for all medical school graduates except individuals in ACGME- or AOA-accredited residency programs. Requires ECFMG certificate from all IMGs for limited permit.
North Carolina	Yes, $25	Yes		Yes, $50	Limited license to resident physicians (ineligible for licensure by endorsement. Limited faculty license for medical school faculty.
North Dakota	Yes, $25				Limited 1-yr license for residents in a clinical program.
Ohio	Yes, $75 (initial) $35 (renewal)	Yes		Yes, $125	Training certificate or full license mandatory for interns, residents, and clinical fellows. Visiting Medical Faculty certificate and Special Activities certificates are $125.
Oklahoma	Yes, $200	Yes	Yes		
Oklahoma DO	NA				
Oregon	Yes, $185	Yes		Yes, $185	
Pennsylvania	Yes, $30			Yes	Graduate license renewal fee is $10.
Pennsylvania DO	Yes, $25				Temporary license for GME valid for up to 12 months.
Puerto Rico	Yes			Yes	Internship/residency licenses to qualified applicants enrolled in an ACGME-accredited residency program who have successfully completed the first part of the medical board examination (basic sciences) or its equivalent (NBME, FLEX, or USMLE).
Rhode Island	Yes, $25	Yes		Yes, $350	Limited medical registration to interns, residents, or fellows. Practice limited to the designated institution and must be under the supervision of a staff physician licensed in this state.
South Carolina	Yes, $150	Yes			Limited licenses for residency programs or limited practices renewable on a yearly basis.
South Dakota	Yes, $50				
Tennessee	Yes	Yes		Yes	

Table 15 (continued)
Teaching (Visiting Professor) and Resident Physician Licenses Issued by State Medical/Osteopathic Boards

	Residents and Prospective Residents			Teaching (Visiting Professor) Licenses	Notes
	Licenses, Permits, Certificates, & Registration	Must Obtain New Permit/License When Changing Residency Programs Within State	Prospective Residents Applying for License Must Have Passed USMLE Step 1		
Tennessee DO	Yes				
Texas	Yes, $50	Yes		Yes, $10 (monthly)	Physician-in-training permits to residents, interns, and fellows (with requirements that gradually increase in difficulty with each renewal)
Utah	Yes				
Vermont	Yes, $40			Yes	Limited license to interns, residents, fellows, or house officers enrolled in ACGME-accredited residency programs and working under supervision of licensed physician at a state-licensed institution or clinic. Physicians appointed full-time to the faculty of the College of Medicine of the Univ of Vermont receive Vermont license, for the duration of the appointment.
Vermont DO	Yes, $40				
Virgin Islands					
Virginia	Yes, $10	Yes		Yes, $125	Limited license for fellowship and teaching positions. Temporary licenses (renewable annually) to interns, residents, and fellows in accredited programs in Virginia.
Washington	Yes, $225			Yes	Limited license to physicians in GME and teaching/research at state institutions and city/county health departments. Teaching (visiting professor) license for teaching/research at state institutions or city/county health fellowships, only to physicians currently licensed in another state or country.
Washington DO	Yes, $225				
West Virginia				Yes, $150	
West Virginia DO	Yes				1-yr limited medical registration for interns
Wisconsin	Yes, $10			Yes, $84	Temporary educational certificates for residency education after first year; may be renewed annually for not more than 4 years.
Wyoming					
Total	**58**	**31**	**10**	**39**	

Note: *All information should be verified with the licensing board; medical licenses are granted to those physicians meeting all state requirements—at the discretion of the board.*

Noneducational Temporary or Limited Licenses, Permits, Certificates, and Registration Issued by State Medical/Osteopathic Boards

Fifty-three boards issue noneducational temporary permits, limited and temporary licenses, or other certificates for the practice of medicine, with fees ranging from zero to $355 (Florida MD board). The terms for the issuance of such certificates vary, but in general they must be renewed once a year with a stipulated maximum number of renewals allowed (usually 5 years). Often, a board will issue a temporary license or permit valid until the next board meeting, at which a candidate's application will be considered.

Some states permit state institutions to hire unlicensed physicians to work under the supervision of licensed physicians. In many instances, the state departments of mental health and public health that operate these hospitals will not hire physicians who have not had at least 1 year of GME in an English-speaking hospital. International medical graduates are generally not considered for these positions unless they are in the United States with a permanent resident visa. An unlicensed physician employed by a state hospital is required in most states to register with the state board of medical examiners, which may issue a limited permit to practice within the institution.

Twenty-six jurisdictions issue locum tenens permits, with fees ranging from zero to $450 (Nevada MD board).

Thirty-one jurisdictions issue inactive licenses (for physicians who want to maintain licensure in that state although they are currently practicing in another state), with fees ranging from zero to $438 (Oregon board).

Thirteen jurisdictions issue retired physicians' licenses, with fees ranging from zero to $125 (New Jersey), and seven issue camp licenses.

Table 16
Noneducational Temporary or Limited Licenses, Permits, Certificates, and Registration Issued by State Medical/Osteopathic Boards

	Noneducational Temporary/Limited Licenses, Permits, and Certificates	Locum Tenens Permits	Inactive Licenses	Retired Physicians' Licenses	Camp Licenses	Additional Notes
Alabama	Yes, $175					Limited license for work in state penal and mental institutions.
Alaska	Yes, $145	Yes	Yes, $225	Yes, $50		Retired physician license: $50 one-time fee
Arizona	Yes	Yes, $200	Yes, $0			
Arizona DO	Yes	Yes, $200				
Arkansas	Yes, $50					
California			Yes	Yes, $0		
California DO			Yes, $150			
Colorado			Yes			
Connecticut	Yes, $150					Temporary permits (valid for 1 year only, not renewable or extendable) only to those physicians who have been offered a position in a state hospital or state facility.
Delaware	Yes, $25		Yes, $142			Temporary permit until board meets to approve candidates
DC			Yes, $120			
Florida	Yes, $355		Yes			
Florida DO	Yes, $100		Yes, $100			
Georgia	Yes, $100		Yes, $140			Temporary permits for reciprocity/endorsement applicants between board meetings
Guam	Yes					
Hawaii	Yes					Not available to physicians against whom disciplinary action is pending in another state.
Idaho	Yes, $100		Yes, $75			Temporary license until next board meeting after application for licensure is complete; no requirements waived.
Illinois	Yes		Yes			
Indiana	Yes, $50	Yes, $50	Yes, $25			
Iowa	Yes, $200		Yes			Temporary license for emergency purposes.
Kansas	Yes, $40		Yes, $100	Yes, $100		Physicians with inactive licenses may not practice medicine in any form, including writing prescriptions.
Kentucky	Yes					Temporary permit until board meets (for endorsement candidates only).
Louisiana	Yes, $0			Yes, $75		
Maine	Yes, $200	Yes	Yes, $400	Yes	Yes, $100	Retired physicians' license for those doing volunteer work; volunteer license is $75
Maine DO	Yes, $0	Yes, $200			Yes, $100	
Maryland			Yes, $50			Physicians with inactive licenses may not practice medicine in any form, including writing prescriptions.
Massachusetts		Yes				
Michigan						
Michigan DO						
Minnesota	Yes, $60			Yes, $50		Temporary license valid until next board meeting at which application is to be considered.

Table 16 (continued)
Noneducational Temporary or Limited Licenses, Permits, Certificates, and Registration Issued by State Medical/Osteopathic Boards

	Noneducational Temporary/Limited Licenses, Permits, and Certificates	Locum Tenens Permits	Inactive Licenses	Retired Physicians' Licenses	Camp Licenses	Additional Notes
Mississippi	Yes				Yes, $25	Ninety-day Youth Camp Permit issued to physicians providing health care only at youth camps approved by the Mississippi State Department of Health.
Missouri	Yes			Yes, $25		
Montana	Yes, $50	Yes	Yes, $100	Yes, $32.50		Thirty-day locum tenens permits available, but candidate must meet all requirements for licensure.
Nebraska		Yes, $0	Yes			
Nevada	Yes	Yes, $450	Yes, $200 (every 2 yrs)			Locum tenens license (one-time only) for 3 months to qualified candidates. Temporary licenses for practice in medically underserved areas (at discretion of the board).
Nevada DO	Yes, $50					
New Hampshire	Yes, $150	Yes, $150			Yes, $75	
New Jersey	Yes			Yes, $125		
New Mexico	Yes, $40		Yes		Yes, $25	
New Mexico DO	Yes, $0					Issued to physicians who have applied for and met licensure requirements between regular board meetings.
New York	Yes					
North Carolina	Yes, $150		Yes			Limited license for practice in medically underserved areas; temporary licenses to eligible endorsement candidates beginning practice prior to board meeting.
North Dakota	Yes, $200	Yes, $200				Locum tenens permit not to exceed 3 months.
Ohio	Yes		Yes	Yes, $0		Limited certificates for employment in state hospitals. Retired physician license: no fee for Emeritus certificate or Volunteer's certificate
Oklahoma	Yes			Yes		Emeritus (may not practice)
Oklahoma DO	NA					
Oregon	Yes, $185		Yes, $438			Locum tenens license limited to 180 days' practice in state in the biennium
Pennsylvania	Yes			Yes		
Pennsylvania DO	Yes					
Puerto Rico	Yes					
Rhode Island	Yes		Yes, $0			
South Carolina	Yes, $75		Yes, $0			Temporary license to any applicant who meets all requirements pending final board approval.
South Dakota		Yes, $50				Sixty-day locum tenens permit.
Tennessee	Yes	Yes	Yes, $50			
Tennessee DO			Yes, $50			
Texas	Yes, $50					Temporary licenses pending final board approval.
Utah			Yes, $50			Inactive license must be renewed every 2 years.
Vermont						

Table 16 (continued)
Noneducational Temporary or Limited Licenses, Permits, Certificates, and Registration Issued by State Medical/Osteopathic Boards

	Noneducational Temporary/Limited Licenses, Permits, and Certificates	Locum Tenens Permits	Inactive Licenses	Retired Physicians' Licenses	Camp Licenses	Additional Notes
Vermont DO	Yes					
Virgin Islands	Yes					Temporary licenses (2 years) for government employment only. Limited-scope inactive licenses (valid 30 days, nonrenewable).
Virginia	Yes		Yes, $130			Temporary license/certificate for continuing education, summer camps, and free clinics.
Washington	Yes			Yes		Temporary permit (valid 90 days) only in conjunction with full application; applicant must have been previously licensed in an approved state.
Washington DO	Yes					
West Virginia	Yes	Yes, $100	Yes, $100		Yes	Temporary license (valid until subsequent board meeting) after completed application for permanent license has been filed, processed, and found in order.
West Virginia DO	Yes					Temporary license granted, at discretion of board, for specific location and need
Wisconsin	Yes, $78	Yes, $153			Yes	Camp physician's license to physicians for locum tenens or for working in a camp for up to 90 days.
Wyoming	Yes, $50					Temporary license between board meetings after completed application for permanent license has been filed, processed, and approved by the board.
Total	**53**	**26**	**31**	**13**	**7**	

Note: All information should be verified with the licensing board; medical licenses are granted to those physicians meeting all state requirements—at the discretion of the board.

Table 16 (continued)
Noneducational Temporary or Limited Licenses, Permits, Certificates, and Registration Issued by State Medical/Osteopathic Boards

Alaska
- Temporary permits for specific period (6 months maximum) after completed application is on file and until board meets to consider permanent licensure.
- Locum tenens permit for 60 days to an MD or DO licensed in another state for purpose of substituting for another Alaska-licensed physician; may extend 3 times.

Arizona
- Locum tenens permit for a 180-day period to a licensed MD who must be sponsored by an Arizona-licensed physician, either MD or DO; issued only once in a 3-year period.

Arkansas
Temporary permits for limited time in emergency or hardship cases, only after application for licensure is complete and waiting to be presented to the board. Valid until next board meeting.

California
- Renewable certificates of registration (awarded on an individual basis) for 1-5 years to physicians who do not immediately meet licensure requirements and who have been offered full-time teaching positions in California medical schools.

Florida
- Temporary Certificate to Practice in Area of Critical Need to MDs with current valid license in another state to practice in Florida communities with a critical need for physicians and a population of less than 7,500.
- Limited License to MDs who meet the same minimum education and training requirements as required for a full medical license and who are retired and have been licensed to practice medicine in any jurisdiction in the United States for at least 10 years. Practice restricted to public agencies or institutions or nonprofit agencies or institutions meeting the requirements of Section 501(c)(3) of the Internal Revenue Code and located in areas of critical medical need.
- A Public Psychiatry Certificate to board-certified psychiatrists who are licensed to practice medicine without restriction in another state and who meet the minimum education and training requirements required for a full medical license. Practice is restricted to a public mental health facility or program funded in part or entirely by state funds.
- A Public Health Certificate to MDs who are graduates of an accredited medical school and hold a master of public health degree or are board-eligible or certified in public health or preventive medicine, or to MDs who are licensed to practice medicine without restriction in another jurisdiction in the United States and hold a master of public health degree or are board eligible or certified in public health or preventive medicine and who meet the minimum education and training requirements required for a full medical license. Practice restricted to employment duties with the Department of Health and Rehabilitative Services.

Hawaii
- Temporary license to physicians working in a state or county agency in conditions of shortage or emergency; and to physicians under the supervision of a licensed MD who plan to take the USMLE exam within 18 months.

Illinois
- Visiting Physician Permits for up to 180 days to persons receiving an invitation or appointment to study, demonstrate, or perform a specific medical, osteopathic, or chiropractic subject or technique in medical, osteopathic, or chiropractic schools; hospitals; or facilities operated pursuant to the Ambulatory Surgical Treatment Center Act.

Indiana
- To physicians holding an active, valid license from another US/Canadian jurisdiction who have applied for and are awaiting board approval of permanent unrestricted license by endorsement of another jurisdiction's valid license; valid for a designated period of 90 days or less.
- To physicians holding a valid, active license from another US/Canadian jurisdiction who are providing health care for a circumscribed period as part of a special program, event, or other activity, including locum tenens; permit valid for up to 30 days and is not renewable.

Kansas
- Temporary permit until next licensure board meeting after application for licensure has been completed, filed, processed, and found to be in order. No temporary permit before passing examination.
- Institutional permits to work in state institutions or mental health centers.
- Out-of-phase special permit.

Kentucky
- Temporary permit until next licensure board meeting after application for licensure has been completed, filed, processed, and found to be in order. No temporary permit before passing examination.

Louisiana
- Unrestricted temporary permits only under extreme circumstances. Board meets every 8 weeks to act on reciprocity licensure applications. Board must act on SPEX applicants requiring unrestricted temporary permit. SPEX applicants issued institutional temporary permit, if necessary, pending results of exam.
- Ninety-day renewable unrestricted permit, pending valid visa issued by the Immigration and Naturalization Service.

Maine
- Temporary (up to 1 year) for duration of community need.
- Licensees not meeting Maine's CME requirements are registered as inactive.

Montana
- Temporary license to physicians for practice in specified location in the interval between board meetings. Board may ask physician to appear at next board meeting for temporary license renewal. No requirements are waived.

Nebraska
- Locum tenens permit for a qualified physician with current license in another state for replacement of a Nebraska physician during a period of temporary leave (maximum of 90 days in any 12-month period).

New Hampshire
- Temporary/restricted license, in the state's best interest. Locum tenens (courtesy license) available to a qualified applicant currently holding an unrestricted active license in another state; valid for a maximum of 100 consecutive days in any 12-month period.

New Jersey
- Temporary license (4 months) for a lawfully qualified physician of another state to take charge of the practice of a licensed New Jersey physician during his or her absence from the state. Exemption from licensure to work in county or state institution for a limited period.

North Dakota
- Temporary license between intervals of board meetings, because an interview is required before a permanent license is issued. Permanent licenses issued only at regularly scheduled meetings (March, July, and November). All licensure requirements must be met and file must be processed completely before a temporary license or locum tenens permit will be issued.

Table 16 (continued)
Noneducational Temporary or Limited Licenses, Permits, Certificates, and Registration Issued by State Medical/Osteopathic Boards

Oklahoma
- Temporary medical licenses during the intervals between board meetings. Candidates for temporary license must meet qualifications for full and unrestricted license. Temporary licenses automatically terminate on the date of the next board meeting, when the applicant may be considered for a full and unrestricted medical license.

Oregon
- Limited License SPEX (LL-SPEX) valid while awaiting results of SPEX examination.
- Limited License-Special (LL-Special) allows applicant with complete file to practice between two board meetings.
- LL-IP good only in state institutions.

Pennsylvania
- Temporary License allows licensee to participate in a medical procedure necessary for the well-being of a specified patient within the Commonwealth or to practice medicine and surgery at a camp or resort for no more than 3 months. Applicants for a temporary license must hold an unrestricted license in another state, territory, possession, or country.
- Extraterritorial License granted to licensed physicians maintaining an office to practice near the boundary line of an adjoining state whose medical practice extends into Pennsylvania.

Puerto Rico
- Public service licenses to qualified applicants who have completed at least 1 year of accredited residency education and who have passed all three parts of the medical board examination or its equivalent (NBME, FLEX, or USMLE).

Note: *All information should be verified with the licensing board; medical licenses are granted to those physicians meeting all state requirements—at the discretion of the board.*

Regulations on the Practice of Telemedicine and Out-of-state Consulting Physicians

For purposes of this publication, *telemedicine* is defined as the delivery of health care services via electronic means from a health care provider in one location to a patient in another. Applications that fall under this definition include the transfer of medical images, such as pathology slides or radiographs, interactive video consultations between patient and provider or between primary care and specialty care physicians, and mental health consultations. Thirty-one states have adopted regulations concerning the practice of telemedicine; eight other states have begun to develop regulations.

Table 17
Regulations on the Practice of Telemedicine and Out-of-state Consulting Physicians

	Practice of Telemedicine		Specific Licensure Restrictions on and/or Requirements for Out-of-state Consulting Physicians
	Has Adopted Regulations	Has Begun to Develop Regulations	
Alabama	Yes		Issues a "special purpose" license (1997)
Alaska			Active Alaska license required. Exceptions are made for an MD or DO who is not a resident of Alaska and who is asked by an Alaskan MD or DO to help in the diagnosis or treatment of a case.
Arizona	Yes		No license required for single or infrequent consultation from out-of-state physician with licensed physician. Full license required of any physician providing services via technology.
Arkansas	Yes		
California MD and DO	Yes		No license required for consultations with a primary care physician licensed in California.
Colorado	Yes		Licensed Colorado physician may consult with physicians licensed in another state. Full license required to use telemedicine to diagnose and treat diseases.
Connecticut	Yes		No license required for any physician residing out of state who is employed to come to Connecticut to render temporary assistance to or consult with a licensed Connecticut physician.
Delaware	Yes		No license required, if physician is licensed in another state and performs a consultation no more than six times a year.
DC		Yes	
Florida	Yes		Physician licensed in another state, territory, or foreign country is permitted to examine the patient, take a history and physical, review laboratory tests and x-rays, and make recommendations about diagnosis and treatment to a licensed Florida physician. The term "consultation" does not include such physician's performance of any medical procedure on or the rendering of treatment to the patient. Full licensure required for out-of-state physicians using telemedicine to treat Florida residents.
Florida DO	Yes		
Georgia	Yes		License required for out-of-state telemedicine.
Guam			Must hold license in state where physician resides.
Hawaii	Yes		Out-of-state consultant must be licensed in the state in which he/she resides; may not open an office (or appoint a place to meet patients or receive calls) in Hawaii.
Idaho			No license required for out-of-state physicians consulted by licensed Idaho physicians. Idaho medical license *is* required if out-of-state physician is directly consulted by an Idaho patient.
Illinois	Yes		Full license required.
Indiana	Yes		
Iowa		Yes	No license required for incidental consultation with out-of-state physicians by licensed Iowa physicians; out-of-state physician must be licensed if providing medical services to Iowa patients.
Kansas	Yes		License required if orders for services are issued for individuals located in Kansas. No license required for consultant licensed in another state who does not open an office or maintain a place to meet patients or receive calls in Kansas. No license required for services performed under supervision or by order of or referral from a licensed Kansas physician.
Kentucky			No license required for single or infrequent consultation from out-of-state physician with licensed physician. Full license required of any physician providing services via technology
Louisiana			
Maine	Yes		No license required for incidental consultation with out-of-state physicians by licensed Maine physicians; out-of-state physician must be licensed if providing medical services to patients in Maine.
Maryland			Maryland license required, unless in consultation with a licensed Maryland physician.
Massachusetts			Full license required.
Michigan		Yes	No license required for a physician living in and authorized to practice in another state or country who, in exceptional circumstances, is called for consultation or treatment by a Michigan health professional.
Minnesota			Cannot assume primary patient care responsibility; physician of record must have Minnesota license; orders are countersigned by licensed Minnesota physician.
Mississippi	Yes		No license required for out-of-state physicians called for consultation by a licensed physician residing in Mississippi. Consultation period cannot exceed 5 days. Full license required for physicians rendering a medical opinion concerning diagnosis or treatment via electronic or other means.

Table 17 (continued)
Regulations on the Practice of Telemedicine and Out-of-state Consulting Physicians

| | Practice of Telemedicine | | |
	Has Adopted Regulations	Has Begun to Develop Regulations	Specific Licensure Restrictions on and/or Requirements for Out-of-state Consulting Physicians
Missouri	Yes		Licensed Missouri physician may consult with physicians licensed in another state. Full license required to use telemedicine to diagnose and treat diseases.
Montana	Yes		License required if an out-of-state consultant establishes a regular, direct physician/patient relationship.
Nebraska	Yes		Nonresident physicians not holding a Nebraska license cannot practice medicine, except when called in consultation by a licensed Nebraska physician.
Nevada	Yes		License required if consultant's work constitutes the practice of medicine.
New Hampshire			License required if consultation is not made directly with a licensed New Hampshire physician or if consulting is more than incidental.
New Jersey		Yes	
New Mexico	Yes		Telemedicine license is required, with some exceptions; contact the Board for more information.
New York		Yes	License in home jurisdiction required.
North Carolina	Yes		North Carolina license required.
North Dakota			North Dakota license required.
Ohio	Yes		Telemedicine license is required, with some exceptions; contact the Board for more information.
Oklahoma	Yes		License required for regular, ongoing treatment; license not required for occasional consultation.
Oregon	Yes		Permanent license required to practice medicine.
Pennsylvania		Yes	Pennsylvania license required.
Puerto Rico			
Rhode Island		Yes	Requirements exist for out-of-state consultants.
South Carolina			Must consult with a licensed South Carolina physician.
South Dakota	Yes		Any nonresident MD or DO who, while located outside South Dakota, provides diagnostic or treatment services through electronic means to a patient in this state under a contract with a health care provider, a clinic in this state that provides health services, or health care facility is engaged in the practice of medicine or osteopathy in South Dakota. Out-of-state MDs or DOs who consult on an irregular basis with a licensed South Dakota physician are not considered to practice in South Dakota.
Tennessee	Yes		Telemedicine license required of out-of-state physicians diagnosing or treating patients in Tennessee. Some exceptions granted.
Texas	Yes		Special Purpose License required for practice of medicine across state lines.
Utah	Yes		No license required of out-of-state physicians consulting with licensed Utah physician; full license required if consulting directly with patient by any means.
Vermont			
Virgin Islands			
Virginia			Virginia license required if practice of medicine occurs in state.
Washington			May not set up an office, appoint a place of meeting patients, or receive calls within this state.
West Virginia	Yes		License required (with exceptions).
West Virginia DO			West Virginia license required
Wisconsin		Yes	
Wyoming	Yes		No license required of physicians residing in and licensed to practice medicine in another state or country called for consultation via telephone, electronic, or any other means by a licensed Wyoming physician. License required if consultations exceed one 7-day period in any 52-week period.
Total	**31**	**8**	

Note: *All information should be verified with the licensing board; medical licenses are granted to those physicians meeting all state requirements—at the discretion of the board.*

Section II.

Medical Licensing Examinations and Organizations

The United States Medical Licensing Examination™ (USMLE)™ *

National Board of Medical Examiners
Philadelphia, Pennsylvania

The United States Medical Licensing Examination (USMLE) is a three-step examination for medical licensure in the United States and is sponsored by the following organizations:

- Federation of State Medical Boards (FSMB)
- National Board of Medical Examiners (NBME)

The Composite Committee, appointed by the FSMB and NBME, governs the USMLE. The Composite Committee establishes rules for the USMLE program. Membership includes representatives from the following:

- FSMB
- NBME
- Educational Commission for Foreign Medical Graduates (ECFMG®)
- American public

In the United States and its territories, the individual medical licensing authorities ("state medical boards") of the various jurisdictions grant a license to practice medicine. Each medical licensing authority sets its own rules and regulations and requires passing an examination that demonstrates qualification for licensure. Results of the USMLE are reported to these authorities for use in granting the initial license to practice medicine. The USMLE provides them with a common evaluation system for applicants for medical licensure. Because individual medical licensing authorities make their own decisions regarding use of USMLE results, licensure applicants should obtain complete information from the licensing authority. Also, the FSMB can provide general information on medical licensure.

The Three Steps of the USMLE: Step 1, Step 2, and Step 3

The USMLE is designed to assess a physician's ability to apply knowledge, concepts, and principles that are important in health and disease and that constitute the basis of safe and effective patient care. The USMLE is a single examination with three steps. Each step is complementary to the others; no step can stand alone in the assessment of readiness for medical licensure.

Step 1 assesses whether medical school students or graduates can understand and apply important concepts of the sciences basic to the practice of medicine, with special emphasis on principles and mechanisms underlying health, disease, and modes of therapy. Step 1 ensures mastery of not only the sciences undergirding the safe and competent practice of medicine in the present, but also of the scientific principles required for maintenance of competence through lifelong learning.

Step 2 assesses whether medical school students or graduates can apply the medical knowledge and understanding of clinical science considered essential for the provision of patient care under supervision, including emphasis on health promotion and disease prevention. The inclusion of Step 2 in the USMLE sequence is intended to ensure that due attention is devoted to principles of clinical science that undergird the safe and competent practice of medicine.

Step 3 assesses whether physicians can apply the medical knowledge and understanding of biomedical and clinical science considered essential for the unsupervised practice of medicine, with emphasis on patient management in ambulatory settings. The inclusion of Step 3 in the USMLE sequence ensures that attention is devoted to the importance of assessing the knowledge of physicians who are assuming independent responsibility for delivering general medical care to patients.

* Portions reprinted with permission from the *USMLE 2003 Bulletin of Information*, copyright © 2002 by the Federation of State Medical Boards of the United States, Inc, and the National Board of Medical Examiners®; and also from the *2001 Annual Report*, copyright © 2002 by the National Board of Medical Examiners.

USMLE Eligibility Requirements and Examination Policies

To be eligible to sit for USMLE Step 1 or Step 2, an applicant must be in one of the following categories at the time of application and on the examination day:

- a medical student officially enrolled in, or a graduate of, a US or Canadian medical school program leading to the MD degree that is accredited by the Liaison Committee on Medical Education (LCME)

- a medical student officially enrolled in, or a graduate of, a United States medical school that is accredited by the American Osteopathic Association (AOA)

- a medical student officially enrolled in, or a graduate of, a medical school outside the United States and Canada and eligible for examination by the ECFMG for its certificate

To be eligible to sit for USMLE Step 3, an applicant must meet all of the following requirements:

- Meet the requirements for taking Step 3 set by the medical licensing authority to which the applicant is applying.

- Obtain the MD degree (or its equivalent) or the DO degree.

- Obtain passing scores on both Steps 1 and 2.

- If a graduate of a medical school outside the United States and Canada, obtain certification by the ECFMG or successfully complete a Fifth Pathway program (see p. 25 for more information).

The USMLE program recommends that, for Step 3 eligibility, licensing authorities require the completion or near completion of at least 1 postgraduate training year in a program of graduate medical education accredited by the Accreditation Council for Graduate Medical Education (ACGME) or the AOA. Applicants should contact the FSMB or the individual licensing authority for complete information on Step 3 eligibility requirements in the state where they plan to be licensed.

Medical students or graduates who plan to take the USMLE must obtain the most recent information from the appropriate registration entity (see page 68) before applying for the examination. See the USMLE Web site at www.usmle.org for updated information.

Computer-based Testing (CBT)

Through CBT, continuous test administration of the USMLE is available to all examinees. Prometric®, part of The Thompson Corporation, provides scheduling and test centers for the USMLE. The Step 1 and Step 2 examinations are administered worldwide; the Step 3 examination is administered only in the United States. To take a USMLE Step, medical students or graduates must meet the eligibility requirements and do the following:

- Obtain application materials from, and then complete and submit the materials to, the appropriate registration entity (see p. 68).

- Receive a Scheduling Permit verifying eligibility and authorizing the applicant to schedule the examination.

- Follow the instructions on the Scheduling Permit to schedule test date(s) at a specific Prometric test center.

- On the scheduled date(s) and at the scheduled time, bring to the Prometric test center the Scheduling Permit and the required identification described on it, and take the test.

Description of the Examinations

The examinations are administered in sessions of eight or nine hours, broken up into sections, or "blocks." The computer keeps track of overall session time, including break time and time allocated for each block of the test. Further information on examination content and sample test materials for all three Steps of the USMLE are available at the USMLE Web site (www.usmle.org).

Step 1

Step 1 has approximately 350 multiple-choice test items, divided into seven 60-minute blocks, administered in one 8-hour testing session.

Step 1 includes test questions in anatomy, behavioral sciences, biochemistry, microbiology, pathology, pharmacology, and physiology; as well as interdisciplinary topics such as nutrition, genetics, and aging. Step 1 is a broadly based, integrated examination. Test questions commonly require examinees to interpret graphic and tabular material, identify gross and microscopic pathologic and normal specimens, and apply basic science knowledge to clinical problems. Step 1 is constructed according to an integrated content outline that organizes basic science material along two dimensions: system and process.

Step 2

Step 2 has approximately 370 multiple-choice test items, divided into eight 60-minute blocks, administered in one 9-hour testing session.

Step 2 includes test questions in internal medicine, obstetrics and gynecology, pediatrics, preventive medicine, psychiatry, surgery, and other areas relevant to provision of care under supervision. The majority of the test questions describe clinical situations and require that examinees provide a diagnosis, prognosis, indication of underlying mechanisms of disease, or the next step in medical care, including preventive measures. Step 2 is a broadly based, integrated examination. Interpretation of tables and laboratory data, imaging studies, photographs of gross and microscopic pathologic specimens, and results of other diagnostic studies is frequently required.

Step 2 is constructed according to an integrated content outline that organizes clinical science material along two dimensions: physician task and disease process.

Step 3

Step 3 has approximately 480 multiple-choice test items, taken in blocks of 35 to 50 items, with 45 to 60 minutes to complete each of these blocks, and approximately nine computer-based case simulations, taken one case in each block, with 15 to 25 minutes to complete each of these blocks.

Step 3 is organized along two principal dimensions: clinical encounter frame and physician task. Step 3 content reflects a data-based model of generalist medical practice in the United States.

Encounter frames capture the essential features of circumstances surrounding physicians' clinical activity with patients. They range from encounters with patients seen for the first time for nonemergency problems, to encounters with regular patients seen in the context of continued care, to patient encounters in (life-threatening) emergency situations. Encounters occur in clinics, offices, nursing homes, hospitals, emergency departments, and on the telephone. Each test item in an encounter frame also represents one of the six physician tasks. For example, initial care encounters emphasize taking a history and performing a physical examination. In contrast, continued care encounters emphasize decisions regarding prognosis and management.

High-frequency, high-impact diseases also organize the content of Step 3. Clinician experts assign clinical problems related to these diseases to individual clinical encounter frames to represent their occurrence in generalist practice.

Step 3 includes Primum® computer-based case simulations (CCS), a test format developed by the NBME that allows the medical student or physician taking the test to provide care for a simulated patient. The test-taker decides which diagnostic information to obtain and how to treat and monitor the patient's progress. The computer records each step taken in caring for the patient and scores overall performance. This format permits assessment of clinical decision-making skills in a more realistic and integrated manner than other available formats.

In Primum CCS, the test-taker may request information from the history and physical examination; order laboratory studies, procedures, and consultants; and start medications and other therapies. Any of the thousands of possible entries that are typed on the "order sheet" are processed and verified by the "clerk." When the test-taker has confirmed that there is nothing further to do, he or she decides when to reevaluate the patient by advancing time. As time passes, the patient's condition changes based on the underlying problem and interventions taken; results of tests are reported and results of interventions must be monitored. The test-taker can suspend the movement of time to consider next steps. While one cannot go back in time, orders can be changed to reflect an updated management plan.

The patient's chart contains, in addition to the order sheet, the reports resulting from orders. By selecting the appropriate chart tabs, the test-taker can review vital signs, progress notes, nurses' notes, and test results. He or she may care for and move the patient among the office, home, emergency department, intensive care unit, and hospital ward.

Preparation for the Examinations

No test preparation courses are affiliated with or sanctioned by the USMLE program. Information on such courses is *not* available from the ECFMG, FSMB, NBME, USMLE Secretariat, or medical licensing authorities.

USMLE Steps are broad in scope and are designed to measure the prospective physician's ability to apply knowledge. The best preparation for the USMLE is a general, thorough review of the content reflected in the descriptions for each Step (available at the USMLE Web site).

A USMLE CD, which contains sample test materials to practice with the testing software, is provided to eligible applicants from their registration entity. The sample test materials are also available at the USMLE Web site. Applicants should run the sample test materials and acquaint themselves with the software well before their test date(s). Practice time is not available on the test day. A brief tutorial on the test day provides a review of the test software, including navigation tools and examination format, prior to beginning the test. It does not provide an opportunity to practice.

Physicians taking Step 3 must practice with the Primum software well in advance of the test. Experience has shown that those who do not practice with the format and mechanics of managing the patients in Primum CCS are likely to be at a disadvantage when taking the cases under standardized test conditions. Extensive practice time is not available on the test day. The CCS software is included on the USMLE CD and at the USMLE Web site.

Examinee Performance on Step 1

Details on the performance of examinees taking Step 1 in 2000 and 2001 are in **Table 18**. Data for 2001 are based upon examinees whose results were reported through January 30, 2002. Approximately 16,400 first-time takers from LCME-accredited US and Canadian medical schools were tested in each of these years. First-time takers from non-US/Canadian medical schools numbered approximately 8,800 and 9,800 for the same years. The pass rates for first-time takers from LCME-accredited US and Canadian medical schools were 93% and 91%, respectively. Because failing examinees generally retake Step 1, the ultimate passing rate across test administrations is expected to increase to approximately 99% for these same examinee groups.

Examinee Performance on Step 2

Details on the performance of examinees taking Step 2 in the 1999-2000 and 2000-2001 academic years are provided in **Table 19**. First-time takers from LCME-accredited US and Canadian medical schools numbered approximately 16,300 and 16,200 for the 1999-2000 and 2000-2001 periods, respectively. First-time takers from non-US/Canadian medical schools numbered approximately 6,100 and 7,100, respectively. The pass rates for first-time takers from LCME-accredited US and Canadian medical schools were 95% both years. As noted with Step 1, given the opportunity to repeat the examination, the ultimate Step 2 passing rate across test administrations is expected to increase to approximately 99% for these same examinee groups.

Examinee Performance on Step 3

Details on the performance of examinees taking Step 3 in 2000 and 2001 are provided in **Table 20**. Data for 2001 are based upon examinees whose results were reported through January 30, 2002. First-time takers who were graduates of

Table 18
2000-2001 USMLE Step 1 Administrations: Number Tested and Percent Passing

	2000		2001*	
	# Tested	% Passing	# Tested	% Passing
US/Canadian Examinees				
LCME Students	18,267	90%	18,380	88%
First-time Takers	16,412	93%	16,368	91%
Repeaters**	1,855	58%	2,012	58%
Osteopathic Students	823	75%	774	69%
First-time Takers	785	77%	723	72%
Repeaters**	38	40%	51	31%
Total US/Canadian	*19,090*	*89%*	*19,154*	*87%*
Non-US/Canadian Examinees				
First-time Takers	8,767	65%	9,835	66%
Repeaters**	4,688	36%	4,259	35%
Total non-US/Canadian	*13,455*	*55%*	*14,094*	*56%*

* Represents data for examinees tested in 2001 and reported through January 30, 2002.

** Repeaters represents examinations given, not number of different examinees.

Table 19
1999-2001 USMLE Step 2 Administrations: Number Tested and Percent Passing

	1999-2000*		2000-2001*	
	# Tested	% Passing	# Tested	% Passing
US/Canadian Examinees				
LCME Students	17,440	93%	17,361	93%
First-time Takers	16,309	95%	16,205	95%
Repeaters**	1,131	66%	1,156	66%
Osteopathic Students	183	90%	300	91%
First-time Takers	178	92%	288	93%
Repeaters**	5	40%	12	42%
Total US/Canadian	*17,623*	*93%*	*17,661*	*93%*
Non-US/Canadian Examinees				
First-time Takers	6,067	70%	7,131	75%
Repeaters**	3,203	41%	3,223	48%
Total non-US/Canadian	*9,270*	*60%*	*10,354*	*66%*

* Data for Step 2 are provided for examinees tested during the period from July 1 to June 30.

** Repeaters represents examinations given, not number of different examinees.

Table 20
2000-2001 USMLE Step 3 Administrations: Number Tested and Percent Passing

	2000		2001*	
	# Tested	% Passing	# Tested	% Passing
US/Canadian Examinees				
LCME Graduates	14,803	92%	14,301	91%
First-time Takers	13,636	95%	13,177	94%
Repeaters**	1,167	61%	1,124	56%
Osteopathic Graduates	62	89%	79	90%
First-time Takers	56	89%	72	89%
Repeaters**	6	83%	7	100%
Total US/Canadian	*14,865*	*92%*	*14,380*	*91%*
Non-US/Canadian Examinees				
First-time Takers	5,471	58%	5,381	61%
Repeaters**	4,533	40%	4,961	40%
Total non-US/Canadian	*10,004*	*50%*	*10,342*	*51%*

* Represents data for examinees tested in 2001 and reported through January 30, 2002.

** Repeaters represents examinations given, not number of different examinees.

LCME-accredited US and Canadian medical schools numbered approximately 13,600 and 13,200 for calendar years 2000 and 2001, respectively. First-time takers who were graduates of non-US/Canadian medical schools numbered approximately 5,500 and 5,400 for the same years. For 2000 and 2001, the pass rates for first-time takers from LCME-accredited US and Canadian medical schools were 95% and 94%, respectively. Like Step 1 and Step 2, the ultimate Step 3 passing rate, accounting for repeat attempts, is expected to increase to approximately 99% for these same examinee groups.

Communicating About USMLE

Complete information on USMLE is available at the USMLE Web site. General inquiries regarding the USMLE or inquires for the USMLE Secretariat may be directed to the NBME or the USMLE Secretariat:

USMLE Secretariat
3750 Market St
Philadelphia, PA 19104-3190
215 590-9700

Contact Information for USMLE

Examination	Type of Applicant	Registration Entity to Contact
Step 1 or Step 2	Students and graduates of medical schools in the US and Canada accredited by the Liaison Committee on Medical Education or the American Osteopathic Association	NBME Applicant Services, 3750 Market St Philadelphia, PA 19104-3190 215 590-9700 215 590-9457 Fax www.nbme.org

Step 1 or Step 2	Students and graduates of medical schools outside the US and Canada	ECFMG
		3624 Market St, Philadelphia, PA 19104-2685
		Application materials:
		    www.ecfmg.org
		    215 375-1913
		    800 500-8249 toll-free in North America
		Other inquiries:
		    215 386-5900
		    215 387-9963 Fax

Step 3	All medical school graduates who have passed Step 1 and Step 2	FSMB Dept of Examination Services 400 Fuller Wiser Rd/Ste 300, Euless, TX 76039-3855 817 868-4041 www.fsmb.org – or – Medical licensing authority

The Federation of State Medical Boards of the United States, Inc.

Founded in 1912, the Federation of State Medical Boards of the United States, Inc (FSMB) is a nonprofit organization composed of the 70 allopathic, osteopathic, and composite medical licensing boards of all the states, the District of Columbia, Guam, Puerto Rico, and the Virgin Islands.

The primary responsibility of each medical licensing board is to protect the public through the regulation of physicians and other health care providers. Within the United States, the organization and activities of each board are determined by state statute, usually referred to as a medical practice act. In general, each state medical board has the authority to license physicians, regulate the practice of medicine, and discipline those who violate the medical practice act.

The FSMB serves as a liaison, advocate, researcher, and educator and information source to the public, to health care organizations, and to state, national, and international authorities. It works to improve the quality, safety, and integrity of US health care by promoting high standards for physician licensure and practice and assisting and supporting state medical boards in regulating medical practice and protecting the public.

FSMB Services

The FSMB provides the following services designed to assist member medical boards in their role as public protectors.

Physician Data Center

A central repository for formal actions taken against physicians by state licensing and disciplinary boards, Canadian licensing authorities, the US armed forces, the US Department of Health and Human Services, and other regulatory bodies, the Data Bank contains more

than 117,000 prejudicial and nonprejudicial actions related to approximately 35,000 physicians. This information is available to licensing and disciplinary boards; military, governmental, and private agencies; and physician credentialing organizations.

Licensure and Assessment Services

In the United States and its territories, a license to practice medicine is a privilege granted only by the individual medical licensing authority of a state or jurisdiction. Each authority sets its own rules and regulations, and each requires successful completion of an examination or certification demonstrating qualification for licensure.

The FSMB, in collaboration with the National Board of Medical Examiners (see p. 73), offers two service packages used by medical licensing authorities for making licensure decisions: The United States Medical Licensing Examination (USMLE™) and the Post-Licensure Assessment System (PLAS).

United States Medical Licensing Examination (USMLE)

The USMLE is a 3-step examination taken by individuals preparing for initial medical licensure in the United States. With steps designed to be taken at different times during medical education and training, the USMLE provides a single pathway for evaluating an individual's ability to apply medical knowledge, concepts and principles to patient care (see p. 62 for more information on USMLE).

Post-Licensure Assessment System (PLAS)

The Post-Licensure Assessment System (PLAS), established in 1998, is a joint program of the FSMB and the National Board of Medical Examiners (NBME). The PLAS provides comprehensive services to medical licensing authorities for use in assessing the ongoing clinical competence of licensed physicians. (More information on PLAS is provided below.)

Federation Credentials Verification Service (FCVS)

The Federation Credentials Verification Service (FCVS) was launched in September 1996 to provide a centralized, uniform process for state medical boards to obtain a verified, primary-source record of a physician's medical credentials. This service is designed to lighten the workload of credentialing staff and reduce duplication of effort by gathering, verifying, and permanently storing the physician's credentials in a central repository at the Federation's offices. FCVS obtains primary source verification of medical education, postgraduate training, examination history, board action history, and identity. This repository of information allows a physician to establish a confidential, lifetime professional portfolio with FCVS which can be forwarded, at the physician's request, to any state medical board that has established an agreement with FCVS—as well as other health care entities.

To request an FCVS application, receive more detailed information about the credentialing process, or request a roster of the state medical boards that accept FCVS documents, call toll-free 888 ASK-FCVS (888 275-3287), access the federation Web site at www.fsmb.org, or send an e-mail to fcvs@fsmb.org.

Legislative Services

The Federation monitors federal and state legislation and regulatory policies that affect medical licensure and discipline. Legislative Services attempts to identify current legislative trends and facilitates communication among member medical boards on issues of mutual interest. Legislative Services assists state medical boards in legislative and administrative efforts to implement Federation policy initiatives through formal policy statements, research assistance, written and oral testimony, letters to legislative leadership, etc. The Federation has played a key role in state and national debates on many prominent issues, including telemedicine, Internet prescribing, physician profiling, management of chronic pain, oversight of resident physicians, managed care, and reduction of medical errors.

Publications

The Federation circulates various publications via print and electronic means to inform the public about medical licensing, regulation, discipline, and medical trends. The guidelines and recommendations for handling key issues—such as telemedicine, pain management, physician profiling, and Internet prescribing—are set forth in published policy documents.

On a quarterly basis, the Federation publishes the *Journal of Medical Licensure and Discipline*, which is distributed to Federation membership, libraries, medical schools, and subscribers around the world. Member boards and their staffs are served by the monthly newsletter *NewsLine* and the online weekly publication *BoardNet News*. An expansive compendium provides detailed information on physician examination and licensing requirements, along with an overview of medical board structure and disciplinary functions.

The Federation also publishes all of its policy documents, organizational updates and the United States Medical Licensing Examination applications, all of which are available online at www.fsmb.org.

Education

The FSMB education department offers various educational programs to its members, including the Annual Meeting, Board Investigator Workshops, Online Seminars, Board Attorney's Workshop, Executive Management Seminar, and New Executives' Orientation. CME and CLE are also available through various program offerings, and the Federation offers a Senior Executive Certification program for its members.

Library Services

The Library Services department provides research assistance to member boards and the general public on topical issues dealing with medical licensure and discipline. Non-member library research requests are based on an hourly charge of $35.

Post-Licensure Assessment System (PLAS)

The Post-Licensure Assessment System (PLAS) is a joint program of the FSMB and the National Board of Medical Examiners (NBME). The PLAS provides comprehensive services to medical licensing authorities for use in assessing the ongoing clinical competence of licensed physicians.

PLAS comprises two independent yet complementary programs: the Special Purpose Examination (SPEX) program and the Assessment Center Program. Collectively, they provide a standardized, national program for assisting state medical boards in ensuring that qualified, competent physicians are licensed to practice medicine.

Special Purpose Examination (SPEX)

The SPEX is a high-quality, objective, and standardized cognitive examination used to assess current knowledge requisite for general, undifferentiated medical practice by physicians who hold or who have held a valid, unrestricted license in a US or Canadian jurisdiction.

SPEX is available to licensing boards for reexamination of physicians for whom the board determines the need for a demonstration of current medical knowledge. SPEX is appropriate for physicians applying for licensure by endorsement who are some years beyond initial examination. SPEX is also frequently used for physicians seeking licensure reinstatement or reactivation after some period of professional inactivity or for a physician involved in a disciplinary proceeding in which the board determines the need for evaluation. Physicians who hold a current, unrestricted license to practice medicine in a US or Canadian jurisdiction are eligible to apply for SPEX as a "self-nominated" candidate, independent of any request or approval from a medical licensing board.

The questions used in SPEX focus on a core of clinical knowledge and relevant underlying basic science principles deemed necessary to form a reasonable foundation for the safe and effective practice of medicine. Specifically, there are two primary dimensions of SPEX: clinical encounter categories (well-care/preventive medicine; acute, circumscribed problems; ill-defined presentations or problems; chronic or progressive illness; emergency conditions, critical care; and behavioral/emotional problems) and physician tasks (data gathering; diagnostic assessment; managing therapy; and applying scientific concepts).

SPEX is a computer-administered examination consisting of 420 multiple-choice questions in two sections of 3 hours and 15 minutes each and is administered through Prometric test centers in coordination with the NBME. Prometric offers test sites across the United States, its territories, Canada, Puerto Rico, and the Virgin Islands. For a more detailed list of testing centers, consult www.prometric.com.

SPEX scores are reported directly to the licensing boards for which SPEX is taken and to the examinee. The FSMB maintains a data bank of all SPEX scores to facilitate interstate endorsement. At the request of the examinee, FSMB will provide certified transcripts of SPEX scores to additional licensing boards.

Assessment Center Program

The PLAS Assessment Program is a multi-tiered service designed to assess a physician's strengths and weaknesses in one or more of the following areas: medical knowledge, clinical reasoning and judgment, communication skills, and patient documentation. Available through the Institute for Physician Evaluation, the PLAS assessment program provides physicians and organizations responsible for licensing and privileging physicians an in-depth analysis of practice skills using state-of-the-art standardized and personalized tools.

Flexible protocols allow for tailoring of an assessment based on the needs of the physician or referral source. Diagnostic information is provided in summary reports that describe performance in qualitative and quantitative formats suitable for designing remedial educational programs of study and training. In some instances, national normative data will be provided for comparison.

Assessment instruments currently include Primum®/ Clinical Case Simulations (a series of uncued computerized patient simulations), standardized practice-friendly multiple-choice question tests (MCQs), and a computerized tool designed to assess clinical judgment. A brief neuropsychologic screening assessment of cognitive skills is also available. As the program evolves, a clinical skills examination will be incorporated into the assessment protocols along with several more personalized assessments, including chart audits and structured clinical interviews. Assessment of the physician in his or her own practice environment through practice audits is also under consideration.

Assessment services will available at regional Institute locations and at more local sites as they become established. In 2002-2003, assessments are expected to be available at centers in Atlanta, Dallas, and Philadelphia.

State medical boards, hospital medical staff review boards, insurers or credentialing organizations, and individuals wishing to self-assess are encouraged to call 888 348-0928 for more details. The Web site www.ipecolorado.org provides more information on the assessment tools, reporting options, and registration and scheduling procedures.

Contact Information

Federation of State Medical Boards of the United States
400 Fuller Wiser Rd/Ste 300
Euless, TX 76039
817 868-4000
817 868-4099 Fax
www.fsmb.org

National Board of Medical Examiners® (NBME®)

The National Board of Medical Examiners (NBME) is an independent, not-for-profit organization that provides high-quality examinations for the health professions. Protection of the health of the public through state-of-the-art assessment is part of the mission of the NBME, along with a major commitment to research and development in evaluation and measurement. The NBME was founded in 1915 to meet the need for a voluntary, nationwide examination that medical licensing authorities could accept as the standard by which to judge candidates for medical licensure. Since that time, it has continued without interruption to provide high-quality examinations for this purpose and has become a model and a resource of international stature in testing methodologies and evaluation in medicine.

NBME Statement of Guiding Principles

The NBME works to protect the health of the public through state-of-the-art assessment of health professionals. While centered on assessment of physicians, this mission encompasses the spectrum of health professionals along the continuum of education, training, and practice and includes research in evaluation as well as development of assessment instruments.

United States Medical Licensing Examination™ (USMLE™)

The USMLE, cosponsored and co-owned by the NBME and the Federation of State Medical Boards (FSMB), is a three-step examination for medical licensure in the United States. Information on the USMLE appears starting on page 62.

Services for Medical Schools and Health Professional Organizations

Through a liaison program with medical schools, the NBME fosters communication between the NBME and medical schools and provides information and assistance to medical educators by producing high-quality assessment tools known as subject examinations. The NBME also provides testing, educational, consultative, and research services to a number of medical specialty boards, societies, and health sciences organizations. Services include developing, administering, and analyzing more than 30 examinations for certification, recertification, in-training, self-assessment, or evaluation of special competence.

For information on these services, visit the NBME Web site at www.nbme.org.

Post-Licensure Assessment

The Post-Licensure Assessment System (PLAS) is a joint activity of the NBME and FSMB and was developed to assist medical licensing authorities in assessing physicians who have already been licensed. The PLAS includes the Special Purpose Examination (SPEX®) and the Assessment Center Program (ACP).

Research and Development

The NBME continually supports intramural research in the fields of clinical skills assessment, advanced methods of testing, and ongoing studies of the validity and reliability of NBME examination programs. In addition, the Edward J. Stemmler Medical Education Research Fund of the NBME assists with extramural research relevant to the mission of the NBME.

NBME Certification and Endorsements

The NBME developed and administered its own three-part examination as part of the National Board Certification Program until it was discontinued with the implementation of the USMLE. Certification was awarded to physicians who

1. received the MD degree from an LCME-accredited medical school;

2. passed at least one NBME Part or Step examination prior to December 31, 1994; and

3. completed, with a satisfactory record, 1 full year (12 months) in a GME program accredited by the Accreditation Council for Graduate Medical Education (ACGME). Accredited internships in Canada were also recognized as meeting this requirement.

Certification by the NBME continues to be used for licensure in the United States for those physicians certified as diplomates prior to implementation of the USMLE and for examinees certified as diplomates who took a combination of NBME and/or USMLE examinations and passed at least one Part or Step prior to December 31, 1994. The last regular administration of Part I occurred in 1991, Part II in April 1992, and Part III in May 1994.

Because some medical students and physicians completed some part of the NBME examination sequence before the implementation of the USMLE, certain combinations of examinations may be considered by medical licensing authorities as comparable to existing examinations. Physicians who passed a combination of examinations should obtain information regarding the acceptability of the combination directly from the medical licensing authority in the jurisdiction where the physician plans to seek licensure.

NBME Certificates and Endorsements

In 2001, the NBME awarded a total of 216 diplomate certificates, and NBME diplomates requested 11,025 endorsements of record of certification to medical licensing authorities.

For further information on NBME certification, contact:

NBME
Applicant Services
3750 Market St
Philadelphia, PA 19104
215 590-9700

NBME Web Site

For further information on the NBME and its programs and services, visit the NBME Web site at www.nbme.org.

National Board of Osteopathic Medical Examiners (NBOME)

Established in 1934, the National Board of Osteopathic Medical Examiners (NBOME) is a not-for-profit corporation dedicated to serving the public and state licensing agencies by administering examinations testing the medical knowledge of those who seek to practice as osteopathic physicians.

The NBOME examinations have been the primary pathway by which osteopathic physicians have applied for licensure to practice osteopathic medicine. A passing score on these examinations verifies a student's adequacy of medical knowledge for practicing osteopathic medicine. Examinations developed by the NBOME are currently accepted in 50 states.

Comprehensive Osteopathic Medical Licensing Examination (COMLEX-USA)

To better assist the state licensing boards in measuring the knowledge required by today's physicians, the NBOME initiated the three-level Comprehensive Osteopathic Medical Licensing Examination (COMLEX-USA) to replace the former three-part NBOME examination series. The COMLEX-USA Level 3 was first administered in February 1995, Level 2 in March 1997, and Level 1 in June 1998.

The COMLEX-USA program is designed to assess the osteopathic medical knowledge considered essential for osteopathic generalist physicians to practice medicine without supervision. COMLEX is constructed in the context of medical problem-solving which involves clinical presentations and physician tasks.

Candidates are expected to utilize the philosophy and principles of osteopathic medicine to solve medical problems. The Clinical Presentation Dimension identifies high-frequency and/or high-impact health issues that osteopathic generalist physicians commonly encounter in practice. The Physician Task Dimension specifies the major steps osteopathic physicians generally undertake in solving medical problems.

Although all three Levels of COMLEX have the same two-dimensional content structure, the depth and emphases of each Level parallel the educational experiences of the candidates. This progressive nature of the COMLEX program ensures the consistency and continuity of the measurement objectives of osteopathic medical licensing examinations.

Level 1

Level 1 emphasizes the medical concepts and principles necessary for understanding the mechanisms of medical problems and disease processes.

Level 1 is a 2-day, written multiple-choice examination covering the basic medical sciences of anatomy, behavioral science, biochemistry, microbiology, osteopathic principles, pathology, pharmacology, physiology, and other relevant areas.

Level 2

Level 2 candidates are expected to demonstrate clinical concepts and principles involved in all steps of medical problem-solving. Level 2 emphasizes the medical concepts and principles necessary for making appropriate medical diagnoses through patient history and physical examination findings.

Level 2 is a 2-day, written multiple-choice examination covering the clinical disciplines of community medicine/medical humanities, emergency medicine, internal medicine, obstetrics/gynecology, osteopathic principles, pediatrics, psychiatry, surgery, and other areas necessary to solve medical problems.

Level 3

Level 3 candidates are expected to demonstrate clinical concepts and principles necessary for solving medical problems as independently practicing osteopathic generalist physicians. Level 3 emphasizes the medical concepts and principles required to make appropriate patient management decisions.

Level 3 is a 2-day, written multiple-choice examination covering the clinical disciplines of community medicine/ medical humanities, emergency medicine, internal medicine, obstetrics/gynecology, osteopathic principles, pediatrics, psychiatry, surgery, and other areas necessary to solve medical problems.

Comprehensive Osteopathic Medical Variable Purpose Examination (COMVEX-USA)

Created by the NBOME, the COMVEX is the newest evaluation instrument offered to osteopathic physicians who need to demonstrate current osteopathic medical knowledge for licensing purposes. It provides the state medical licensing boards a clear evaluation of a candidate's knowledge of current osteopathic medical practices.

The COMVEX is available to candidates through the individual state licensing boards.

Contact Information

National Board of Osteopathic Medical Examiners, Inc.
8765 W Higgins Rd/Ste 200
Chicago, IL 60631-4101
773 714-0622
773 714-0631 Fax
www.nbome.org

Section III.

Information for International Medical Graduates

Educational Commission for Foreign Medical Graduates (ECFMG®)

Stephen S. Seeling, JD
Vice President for Operations
Educational Commission for Foreign Medical Graduates
Philadelphia, Pennsylvania

The Educational Commission for Foreign Medical Graduates (ECFMG®*), through its program of certification, assesses the readiness of international medical graduates to enter residency or fellowship programs in the United States that are accredited by the Accreditation Council for Graduate Medical Education (ACGME).

The ECFMG and its sponsoring organizations define an international medical graduate (IMG) as a physician who received his/her basic medical degree or qualification from a medical school located outside of the United States and Canada. The physician's medical school and graduation year must be listed in the *International Medical Education Directory* (*IMED*) of the Foundation for Advancement of International Medical Education and Research (FAIMER^SM). The FAIMER *IMED* is available on the ECFMG Web site at www.ecfmg.org. US citizens who have completed their medical education in schools outside of the United States and Canada are considered IMGs; non-US citizens who have graduated from medical schools in the United States and Canada are not considered IMGs.

ECFMG certification assures directors of ACGME-accredited residency and fellowship programs, and the people of the United States, that IMGs have met minimum standards of eligibility required to enter such programs. ECFMG certification does not, however, guarantee that such graduates will be accepted into these programs, since the number of applicants often exceeds the number of available positions.

ECFMG certification is one of the eligibility requirements to take Step 3 of the United States Medical Licensing Examination (USMLE). Most states in the United States also require ECFMG certification to obtain licensure to practice medicine.

---

* The terms "ECFMG" and "CSA" are registered in the US Patent and Trademark Office.

ECFMG Certification Requirements

To be eligible for ECFMG certification, international medical graduates must meet the following requirements:

Examination Requirements

1. Pass the basic medical and clinical science components of the medical science examination within a 7-year period.** USMLE Step 1 (basic medical) and Step 2 (clinical) are the examinations currently administered that meet this requirement.

ECFMG accepts a passing performance on former medical science examinations for the purpose of ECFMG certification; those formerly administered by ECFMG are:

- ECFMG Examination
- Visa Qualifying Examination (VQE)
- Foreign Medical Graduate Examination in the Medical Sciences (FMGEMS)
- Part I and Part II Examinations of the National Board of Medical Examiners (NBME)

Combinations of exams are also acceptable. Specifically, applicants who have passed only part of the former VQE, FMGEMS, or the NBME Part I or Part II may combine a passing performance on the basic medical science component of one of these exams or USMLE Step 1 with a passing performance on the clinical science component of one of the other exams or USMLE Step 2, provided that the components are passed within the period specified for the exam program. Additionally, ECFMG accepts, for the

---

** This policy applies only to ECFMG certification. The USMLE program has made specific recommendations to medical licensing authorities regarding the time to complete all three Steps and the number of attempts allowed to pass each Step. Applicants who are taking the Steps for the purpose of licensure should refer to *Time Limit and Number of Attempts Allowed to Complete All Steps, Formerly Administered Examinations* and *Retakes* in the USMLE *Bulletin of Information* for more information. Applicants should also contact the medical licensing authority of the jurisdiction where they plan to apply for licensure or the FSMB, since licensure requirements vary among jurisdictions.

purpose of its certification, a score of 75 or higher on each of the 3 days of a single administration of the former Federation Licensing Examination (FLEX), if taken prior to June 1985.***

2. Pass the English language proficiency test. Applicants can satisfy this requirement by achieving a score acceptable to ECFMG on the Test of English as a Foreign Language (TOEFL) and requesting that ECFMG accept the TOEFL score in fulfillment of this requirement. A passing performance on the former ECFMG English Test is also accepted by ECFMG to meet the English language proficiency requirement for ECFMG certification. Passing performance on either test is valid for 2 years from the date passed for the purpose of entry into graduate medical education.

3. Pass the Clinical Skills Assessment (CSA®*). The CSA is a 1-day exam that requires examinees to demonstrate both clinical proficiency and spoken English language proficiency. The CSA is administered by ECFMG throughout the year. Passing performance on the CSA is valid for 3 years from the date passed for the purpose of entry into graduate medical education.

Medical Education Credential Requirements

4. Document the completion of all requirements for, and receipt of, the final medical diploma. The physician's medical school and graduation year must be listed in the *International Medical Education Directory* (*IMED*). All IMGs must have had at least 4 credit years (academic years for which credit has been given toward completion of the medical curriculum) in attendance at a medical school listed in *IMED*. ECFMG requires all applicants for certification to submit the final medical diploma. All documents provided to ECFMG are sent for verification to appropriate officials of the medical schools that issued the documents.

The *Directory* is available on the ECFMG Web site at www.ecfmg.org. The *Directory* was developed and is

*** This policy applies only to ECFMG certification. Use of the former FLEX components or the former NBME parts to fulfill eligibility requirements for Step 3 is no longer accepted. Applicants taking the Steps for the purpose of licensure should refer to *Formerly Administered Examinations* in the USMLE *Bulletin of Information*. Applicants should also contact the medical licensing authority of the jurisdiction where they plan to apply for licensure or the FSMB for specific information on licensure requirements.

maintained by the Foundation for Advancement of International Medical Education and Research (FAIMERSM), a nonprofit foundation of the ECFMG. The *Directory* contains information supplied by countries about their medical schools. FAIMER is not an accrediting agency.

Standard ECFMG Certificate

The ECFMG issues the Standard ECFMG Certificate to applicants who meet all of the examination and medical education credential requirements. Applicants must also pay any outstanding charges on their ECFMG financial accounts before their certificates are issued. Standard ECFMG Certificates are sent approximately 2 weeks after all of these requirements have been met.

A Standard ECFMG Certificate includes

- the name of the applicant;
- the applicant's USMLE/ECFMG Identification Number;
- the dates that examination requirements were met;
- the date that the certificate was issued;
- the date through which the passing performance on the English test remains valid for the purpose of entry into graduate medical education; and,
- the date through which the passing performance on the CSA remains valid for the purpose of entry into graduate medical education.

Certificate Revalidation Policy

Two of the exam dates on the Standard ECFMG Certificate are subject to expiration for the purpose of entering graduate medical education programs. The English test date is valid for 2 years from the most recent date of passing performance. The Clinical Skills Assessment date is valid for 3 years from the most recent date of passing performance. If the English test date has expired, an applicant will be required to demonstrate a performance acceptable to the ECFMG on the TOEFL exam before entering a graduate medical education program. If the CSA date has expired, an applicant will be required to pass a subsequent CSA before entering a graduate medical education program. Once these exam requirements are met, a revalidation sticker for the appropriate examination is sent to the applicant to be affixed to the Standard ECFMG Certificate. Each revalidation sticker is unique to the individual applicant and includes the same identification number that is on the Standard ECFMG Certificate.

If an applicant's English test/CSA date(s) expire before the applicant's Standard ECFMG Certificate is issued, the applicant may revalidate these dates, as described above, prior to becoming certified by ECFMG. In this event, the English test/CSA valid-through date(s) on the Standard ECFMG Certificate will reflect the applicant's most recent passing performances on these exams.

After an applicant enters an ACGME-accredited program of graduate medical education in the United States, the applicant can request permanent validation of the Standard ECFMG Certificate. This means that the English test and CSA dates are no longer subject to expiration. To request permanent validation, the applicant and an authorized official of the training institution must complete the *Request for Permanent Validation of Standard ECFMG Certificate* (Form 246) and send it to ECFMG. After ECFMG receives and verifies the information contained on the form, a sticker indicating *valid indefinitely* status will be mailed to the applicant to be affixed to the Standard ECFMG Certificate. Each permanent validation sticker is unique to the individual applicant and includes the same identification number that is on the Standard ECFMG Certificate.

Medical Science Examination

The ECFMG requires a passing score on both a basic medical science test and a clinical science test to meet the medical science examination requirement for ECFMG certification. Step 1 (basic medical) and Step 2 (clinical) of the USMLE are the exams currently administered that meet this requirement.

Step 1 and Step 2 of the USMLE

The USMLE is a single, three-step exam for medical licensure in the United States that provides a common system to evaluate applicants for medical licensure. The USMLE is sponsored by the Federation of State Medical Boards of the United States (FSMB) and the NBME. The USMLE is governed by a committee consisting of members of the FSMB, NBME, ECFMG, and the American public. The USMLE Steps 1, 2, and 3 replaced FLEX and the NBME Parts I, II, and III.

The ECFMG determines whether international medical students/graduates are eligible to take USMLE Step 1 and Step 2 and registers eligible applicants to take these exams for the purpose of ECFMG certification. The NBME registers eligible students/graduates of US and Canadian medical schools accredited by the Liaison Committee on Medical Education or the American Osteopathic Association to take Step 1 and Step 2.

The USMLE is administered by computer. Prometric, Inc®, a subsidiary of Thomson Learning™, provides scheduling and test centers for the USMLE. Step 1 and Step 2 are delivered throughout the year at Prometric Test Centers worldwide.

Table 21 shows the performance of IMGs for recent administrations of Step 1 and Step 2.

English Language Proficiency Test

Physicians who assume patient care responsibilities in graduate medical education programs in the United States must be proficient in the English language. Proficiency in English is also one of the requirements for obtaining a visa to enter the United States. As a result, applicants for ECFMG certification are required to demonstrate competence in the English language.

Table 21
Examinee Performance for International Medical Graduates/Students Taking
USMLE Step 1 and Step 2 Examinations

	USMLE Step 1 January 1, 2001 - December 31, 2001			USMLE Step 2 July 1, 2000 - June 30, 2001		
	Number of Administrations	Number Passing	Percent Passing	Number of Administrations	Number Passing	Percent Passing
Total	14,055	7,923	56%	10,355	6,867	66%
First-time Takers	9,784	6,432	66%	7,096	5,304	75%
Repeaters	4,271	1,491	35%	3,259	1,563	48%
US Citizens	3,352	1,545	46%	2,530	1,618	64%
First-time Takers	1,954	1,081	55%	1,703	1,231	72%
Repeaters	1,398	464	33%	827	387	47%
Foreign Citizens	10,703	6,378	60%	7,825	5,249	67%
First-time Takers	7,830	5,351	68%	5,393	4,073	76%
Repeaters	2,873	1,027	36%	2,432	1,176	48%

Notes: Step 1 First-time Takers are those examinees with no prior Step 1 and no prior NBME Part I examinations.

Step 2 First-time Takers are those examinees with no prior Step 2 and no prior NBME Part II examinations.

Citizenship for both Step 1 and Step 2 is as of the time of entrance into medical school.

To satisfy the English language proficiency requirement for ECFMG certification, applicants must achieve a score acceptable to ECFMG on the Test of English as a Foreign Language (TOEFL). The TOEFL score submitted to fulfill this requirement must be for a TOEFL exam taken within 2 years of the date that the applicant's request for TOEFL score acceptance is received at ECFMG. Applicants who passed the former ECFMG English Test (administered for the last time on March 3, 1999) may use their passing performance on this exam to satisfy the requirement.

The TOEFL is offered throughout the world by the Educational Testing Service® (ETS®). For information and application materials for the TOEFL exam, contact:

Educational Testing Service
Princeton, NJ 08541
609 771-7100
E-mail: toefl@ets.org
www.toefl.org

Applicants who take the TOEFL exam to fulfill the English language proficiency requirement should refer to *Test of English as a Foreign Language (TOEFL)* in the ECFMG *Information Booklet* for information on the minimum score that the ECFMG will accept and instructions on how to have the ECFMG evaluate their TOEFL score.

Clinical Skills Assessment

The Clinical Skills Assessment (CSA) evaluates an examinee's ability to gather and interpret clinical patient data and communicate effectively in English. The CSA consists of 11 testing stations, 10 of which are scored; in each station examinees encounter a Standardized Patient (SP), a lay person trained to realistically and consistently portray a patient. The SPs respond to questions from examinees with answers appropriate to the patient being portrayed and react appropriately to physical examination maneuvers. Examinees are expected to proceed through each encounter with an SP as they would with a real patient.

The CSA assesses whether an examinee can obtain a relevant medical history, perform a focused physical examination, and compose a written record of the patient encounter. The CSA also requires examinees to demonstrate proficiency in *spoken* English and appropriate interpersonal skills, as evaluated by the Standardized Patients encountered in the test stations.

The ECFMG administered over 7,000 assessments from February 1, 2001, through January 31, 2002. Approximately 80% of those taking CSA during this period received passing results.

Standard ECFMG Certificates Issued in 2001

During 2001, 5,934 Standard ECFMG Certificates were issued. Table 22 shows the distribution of recipients of Standard ECFMG Certificates by country of medical school and citizenship. In 2001, medical schools in India and Dominica had the largest number of recipients: 1,194 (20.1%) were graduates of Indian medical schools and 433 (7.3%) of the recipients received their medical degrees in Dominica.

Based upon country of citizenship, citizens of the United States formed the largest group of recipients. Of the certificates issued in 2001, 1,518 (25.6%) were to US citizens. Citizens of India were the second largest group with 1,165 (19.6%) recipients.

Electronic Residency Application Service (ERAS®)

Most residency programs require applicants to apply through the Electronic Residency Application Service (ERAS), which was developed by the Association of American Medical Colleges. ERAS transmits residency applications and supporting documents to residency program directors over the Internet. The ECFMG serves as the designated Dean's Office for international medical students and graduates applying to residency programs through ERAS.

Table 22
Standard ECFMG Certificates Issued in 2001: Distribution of Recipients by Country of Medical School and Citizenship

Country	Country of Medical School*		Country of Citizenship	
	Number	%	Number	%
Canada	0	0.0	102	1.7
China	147	2.5	151	2.5
Colombia	108	1.8	98	1.7
Dominica	433	7.3	2	0.0
Dominican Republic	107	1.8	14	0.2
Egypt	90	1.5	82	1.4
Germany	126	2.1	97	1.6
Grenada	372	6.3	4	0.1
Hungary	55	0.9	10	0.2
India	1,194	20.1	1,165	19.6
Iran	102	1.7	148	2.5
Ireland	86	1.4	23	0.4
Israel	102	1.7	24	0.4
Jordan	46	0.8	51	0.9
Lebanon	104	1.8	118	2.0
Mexico	81	1.4	45	0.8
Montserrat	196	3.3	0	0.0
Netherlands Antilles	109	1.8	0	0.0
Nigeria	113	1.9	110	1.9
Pakistan	407	6.9	368	6.2
Philippines	218	3.7	147	2.5
Poland	77	1.3	38	0.6
Romania	115	1.9	108	1.8
Russia	109	1.8	76	1.3
Syria	112	1.9	113	1.9
United Kingdom	70	1.2	84	1.4
USA	0	0.0	1,518	25.6
USSR	0	0.0	59	1.0
Countries with fewer than 50 recipients	1,255	21.1	1,179	19.9
Total	5,934	100.0	5,934	100.0

Notes:

Citizenship is as of the time of entrance into medical school.

* For country of medical school, the countries of the former USSR are represented separately.

Percentages may not total 100% due to rounding.

Specialties utilizing ERAS 2003 (for residency positions beginning in July 2003) are:

- Anesthesiology
- Dermatology
- Diagnostic Radiology
- Emergency Medicine
- Family Practice
- Family Practice/Physical Medicine and Rehabilitation combined programs
- Internal Medicine (Preliminary and Categorical)
- Internal Medicine/Emergency Medicine combined programs
- Internal Medicine/Family Practice combined programs
- Internal Medicine/Pediatrics combined programs
- Internal Medicine/Physical Medicine and Rehabilitation combined programs
- Internal Medicine/Psychiatry combined programs
- Nuclear Medicine
- Obstetrics/Gynecology
- Orthopedic Surgery
- Pathology
- Pediatrics
- Pediatrics/Emergency Medicine combined programs
- Pediatrics/Physical Medicine and Rehabilitation combined programs
- Pediatrics/Psychiatry/Child and Adolescent Psychiatry combined programs
- Physical Medicine and Rehabilitation
- Plastic Surgery (GY1)
- Psychiatry
- Radiation Oncology
- Surgery
- Transitional Year
- Urology
- All US Army and Navy programs

Additional specialties are expected to use ERAS for residency programs beginning in July 2004. Information on participating specialties for ERAS 2004 will be posted on the ERAS home page of the ECFMG Web site as it becomes available. Applicants should contact residency program directors for specific requirements and deadlines.

To obtain an ERAS application materials request form and specific information on ERAS, applicants should visit the ECFMG web site at www.ecfmg.org/eras. Applicants may also contact:

ECFMG ERAS Program
PO Box 11746
Philadelphia, PA 19101-1746
E-mail: eras-support@ecfmg.org
215 386-5900
215 222-5641 Fax

Visas

To obtain a visa to enter the United States to perform services as members of the medical profession or to receive graduate medical education, certain alien physicians are required, under the provisions of Public Law 94-484, to pass NBME Part I and Part II examinations or an examination determined to be equivalent for this purpose. The Secretary of Health and Human Services has recognized USMLE Step 1 and Step 2 as well as the former Visa Qualifying Examination (VQE) and the Foreign Medical Graduate Examination in the Medical Sciences (FMGEMS) as equivalent to NBME Part I and Part II examinations for the purposes of PL 94-484. To obtain additional information on visa requirements, foreign national physicians should refer to the Exchange Visitor Sponsorship Program home page of the ECFMG Web site at www.ecfmg.org/evsp, US Embassies or Consulates abroad, or the US Immigration and Naturalization Service.

Exchange Visitor Sponsorship Program

The ECFMG is authorized by the United States Department of State (DOS) to sponsor foreign national physicians as J-1 Exchange Visitors in accredited graduate medical education or training programs. The objectives of this program are to enhance international exchange in the field of medicine and to promote mutual understanding between the people of the United States and other countries through the interchange of persons, knowledge, and skills.

Table 23
Exchange Visitor Sponsorship Program for Physicians:
Number of J-1 Physicians in Graduate Medical Education
Programs in the United States, July 1, 2000, to June 30, 2001

Specialty	Count
ACGME-accredited Programs	
Allergy and Immunology	47
Anesthesiology	630
Colon and Rectal Surgery	12
Dermatology	21
Emergency Medicine	24
Family Practice	230
Internal Medicine	4,138
Medical Genetics	14
Neurological Surgery	55
Neurology	367
Nuclear Medicine	17
Obstetrics and Gynecology	107
Ophthalmology	76
Orthopedic Surgery	52
Otolaryngology	29
Pathology - Anatomic and Clinical	334
Pediatrics	885
Physical Medicine and Rehabilitation	49
Plastic Surgery	25
Preventive Medicine	4
Psychiatry	597
Radiation Oncology	22
Radiology - Diagnostic	280
Surgery - General	490
Thoracic Surgery	69
Transitional Year	28
Urology	33
ABMS Board-approved Combined Programs	
Internal Medicine/Neurology	4
Internal Medicine/Pediatrics	41
Internal Medicine/Physical Medicine and Rehabilitation	3
Internal Medicine/Preventive Medicine	1
Internal Medicine/Psychiatry	8
Pediatrics/Emergency Medicine	1
Pediatrics/Physical Medicine and Rehabilitation	1
Pediatrics/Psychiatry/Child and Adolescent Psychiatry	1
Total	**8,695**

The program is administered by ECFMG in accordance with the provisions set forth in an agreement between ECFMG and the DOS and the federal regulations established to implement the Mutual Educational and Cultural Exchange Act. ECFMG is responsible for ensuring that all Exchange Visitor Physicians and host institutions comply with the federal requirements for participation. ECFMG issues a Certificate of Eligibility for Exchange Visitor J-1 Status (Form IAP-66) for qualified applicants. This document must be processed through the United States Embassy or Consulate and the Immigration and Naturalization Service (INS) to secure the J-1 visa.

The Federal regulations refer to Exchange Visitor Physicians seeking J-1 sponsorship in accredited clinical programs as *alien physicians*. These applicants must meet the following general requirements:

- Pass USMLE Step 1 and Step 2 or the former VQE, NBME Part I and Part II, or FMGEMS (*Note:* The former 1-day ECFMG Examination does not meet the requirements for J-1 visa sponsorship.);

- Hold a valid Standard ECFMG Certificate (Graduates of LCME- and AOA-accredited US and Canadian medical schools are not required to be ECFMG-certified.);

- Hold a contract or an official letter of offer for a position in an accredited graduate medical education or training program that is affiliated with a medical school;

- Provide a statement of need from the Ministry of Health of the country of nationality or last legal permanent residence. This statement must provide written assurance that the country needs specialists in the area in which the Exchange Visitor will receive training and that he/she will return to the country upon completion. (*Note:* If permanent residence is in a country other than that of citizenship, the Ministry of Health letter must come from the country of last legal permanent residence.)

The duration of stay for a J-1 Exchange Visitor Physician is limited to the time typically required to complete the advanced medical education program. This refers to the specialty and subspecialty certification requirements published by the American Board of Medical Specialties (ABMS). Participation is further limited to 7 years and is reserved for those progressing in approved training programs.

J-1 Exchange Visitor Physicians sponsored for participation in nonclinical programs primarily involved with observation, consultation, teaching, or research are categorized as research scholars. Unlike alien physicians, participants in these programs generally do not have to pass US medical licensing or English examinations and are not required to be ECFMG-certified. Research scholars are limited to activities involving no patient contact or only incidental patient contact. The maximum period of participation for research scholars is 3 years.

Table 23 shows that the ECFMG sponsored 8,695 Exchange Visitor Physicians in US graduate medical education programs for the academic year July 1, 2000, to June 30, 2001. In the alien physician category, the ECFMG sponsored 5,201 in clinical residency (specialty) programs and 3,428 in clinical fellowships (subspecialty training) in 2000-2001. A total of 66 foreign nationals were sponsored in the research scholar category. Consistent with past trends, foreign nationals from India, Pakistan, and the Philippines represented a major segment (35%) of ECFMG-sponsored J-1 physicians for this period.

For application materials and specific information on ECFMG sponsorship, applicants should visit the ECFMG Web site at www.ecfmg.org/evsp. Applicants may also contact:

Educational Commission for Foreign Medical Graduates
Exchange Visitor Sponsorship Program
PO Box 41673
Philadelphia, PA 19101-1673
215 823-2121
215 386-9766 Fax

Certification Verification Service (CVS)

The ECFMG's Certification Verification Service provides primary source confirmation of the ECFMG certification status of IMGs. The Joint Commission on Accreditation of Healthcare Organizations (JCAHO) has determined that an accredited health organization will satisfy the Joint Commission requirement for primary source verification of medical school completion for IMGs if it confirms directly with the ECFMG that an applicant possesses a valid Standard ECFMG Certificate.

The ECFMG will confirm an applicant's certification status when a request is received in writing from a medical licensing authority, residency program director, hospital, or other organization that, in the judgment of ECFMG, has a legitimate interest in such information. For status reports sent to medical licensing authorities, the request can also be sent to ECFMG by the applicant. Requesting organizations must normally secure and retain the applicant's signed authorization to obtain certification information. Please note that there may be a fee for this service.

Requests for confirmation must contain the applicant's name, date of birth, and USMLE / ECFMG Identification Number, as well as the name and address of the organization to which the confirmation should be sent. Confirmations are mailed to the requesting organization within approximately 2 weeks. Confirmations are not sent to applicants directly.

For individuals who apply to residency programs through ERAS, the ECFMG automatically sends an electronic ECFMG status report at the time that their applications are processed to all of the programs to which they applied. If an applicant's ECFMG certification status changes during the ERAS application process, the ECFMG will automatically send an updated status report to all programs to which the applicant applied.

To obtain the appropriate request form(s) and additional information, refer to the CVS home page on the ECFMG web site at www.ecfmg.org/cvs or contact:

Educational Commission for Foreign Medical Graduates
CVS Department
PO Box 13679
Philadelphia PA 19101-3679
215 386-5900

Contact Information

Interested individuals can access the ECFMG *Information Booklet* and apply online for USMLE Step 1 and Step 2 and the ECFMG CSA by visiting the ECFMG Web site at www.ecfmg.org. The ECFMG Web site also provides access to important updates, ECFMG's online services, and more than 50 ECFMG publications and forms.

Individuals who do not have access to the Internet may request a copy of the ECFMG *Information Booklet* and application materials by calling:

- 800 500-8249, toll-free, from within North America, or
- 215 375-1913, from any location worldwide.

For requests by fax or mail or for specific inquiries, contact the ECFMG at:

ECFMG
3624 Market St
Philadelphia, PA 19104-2685
215 386-5900
215 387-9963 Fax

Immigration Overview for International Medical Graduates

Robert D. Aronson is a partner in the immigration law firm of Ingber & Aronson, which practices exclusively in the area of immigration and nationality law. The major area of his practice deals with immigration matters for foreign physicians and US medical institutions nationwide. He served as an Immigration Consultant to the Council on Graduate Medical Education (COGME) of the US Department of Health and Human Services and is a member of the Liaison Committee of his professional association, the American Immigration Lawyers Association to the US Department of State. Mr. Aronson was previously a Fulbright Fellow at the law schools of Harvard University and Moscow State University.

Introduction

This article outlines current immigration laws and policies that affect the physician community. This particular area of the law has become extremely complex owing to the continuing rapid changes within both the immigration and medical reform movements, as well as the aftermath of September 11. What is becoming more clear is that IMGs can be an appropriate source for serving the needs of certain vulnerable patient populations, including rural, minority, ethnic, and low-income patients, and, in this regard, our immigration laws have developed certain special procedures to facilitate the relocation of foreign physicians to traditionally hard-to-fill placements.

Immigration Law Overview

All foreign nationals enter the United States in one of two broad immigration categories-either under a temporary, nonimmigrant visa or as a permanent resident. There are comparative advantages to both these categories. In the case of the temporary, nonimmigrant visa classifications, it is usually possible to gain this type of immigration coverage in a relatively short period of time. The two most common temporary, nonimmigrant classifications used by

IMGs are the J-1 Exchange Visitor program and the H-1B Temporary Worker classification. Both these classifications, however, limit a physician's duration of residence in the United States and impose strict controls over the range of employment authorization, although they do have the advantage of being relatively quick to obtain. In contrast, permanent residence provides a foreign national with both an unlimited duration of residence and full, unrestricted employment authorization, although the processing time is much greater.

Temporary, Nonimmigrant Classifications

Most IMGs in graduate medical education (GME) programs arrive under the J-1 Exchange Visitor program. This program is administered by the US Department of State (DOS) and is intended to provide a broad range of foreign nationals with educational, employment, and training opportunities in the United States.

An IMG applying for a J-1 visa must first obtain certification from the Educational Commission for Foreign Medical Graduates (ECFMG), the implementing agency for the J-1 Exchange Visitor program for physicians. To earn an ECFMG Certificate, an IMG must

1. pass stipulated examinations so as to establish medical competence, which at present consists solely of the United States Medical Licensing Examination (USMLE), Steps 1 and 2;

2. pass the ECFMG English language examination to establish English language competence;

3. possess an MD from a foreign medical school listed in the *World Directory of Medical Schools*, published by the World Health Organization.

All J-1 trainees must receive ECFMG certification (Canadian medical school graduates are exempt from this requirement, because Canadian medical education and training are accredited under US standards).

Upon entry to the United States, an IMG is authorized to pursue GME for a period of up to 7 years to achieve stipulated training objectives. Each year, the GME program, in conjunction with the IMG, needs to file an extension application with the ECFMG. Extensions beyond this 7-year limit may be granted only upon a showing of "extraordinary circumstances."

Without exception, all J-1 physicians in clinical training are subject to a mandatory 2-year home residence obligation, regardless of country of citizenship or last permanent residence. In order for an IMG to ultimately qualify for permanent residence, he/she needs to either return to his/her home country for a 2-year period or obtain a waiver of this 2-year obligation.

By law, a waiver of this obligation is available only on the basis of the following three grounds:

- if the J-1 physician will suffer from persecution in his/her home country or country of last permanent residence;

- if fulfillment of the 2-year home residence obligation will subject a US citizen spouse or child to exceptional hardship; or

- based upon a recommendation issued by a government agency interested in the physician's continued residence/employment in the United States.

Without question, the vast majority of J-1 physicians who receive waivers do so on the basis of recommendations issued by government agencies. Generally speaking, such waivers fall within four basic patterns:

- employment by a federal agency, such as the Department of Veterans Affairs;

- recognition of outstanding academic and research achievements, as determined by the Department of Health and Human Services;

- service to medically underserved patient populations, particularly in rural communities;

- pursuant to the sponsorship of a state Department of Health, under recent legislation that authorizes each state to sponsor up to 20 IMGs per year for waivers of their home residence obligation.

Rather than using the J-1 Exchange Visitor program, with its 2-year home residence requirement, an increasing number of foreign physicians are entering the United States under the H-1B Temporary Worker provisions. This visa classification enables a foreign national to enter the United States to accept professional-level employment for a period of up to 6 years. In most instances, H-1B coverage can be obtained within roughly 60-90 days.

In order for an IMG to qualify for H-1B benefits, all of the following four criteria must be met:

- possession of a full, unrestricted state medical license or the "appropriate authorization" for the position;

- an MD degree or a full unrestricted foreign license;

- English language competence as established either through graduation from an accredited medical school or by passing the ECFMG English language exam;

- the Federation Licensing Examination (FLEX) or its equivalents—the National Board of Medical Examiners (NBME), Parts I, II, and III, or the USMLE, Steps 1, 2, and 3.

As a result of this FLEX equivalency issue, many Canadian physicians do not qualify for H-1B benefits. The standard Canadian medical credential—the Licentiate of the Medical Council of Canada (LMCC)—is widely accepted among the states for medical licensure. Therefore, most Canadian physicians have traditionally not had any reason to sit for the FLEX or its stipulated equivalents. In this manner, H-1B immigration requirements have established different credentialing standards from those of the state medical licensure boards, which have traditionally been the primary judge of physician competence.

Permanent Residence Strategies

There are various ways for a foreign national to qualify for permanent residence, ranging from familial relationships with US citizens or permanent residents to fear of persecution so as to merit refugee entitlement. In most instances, though, an IMG will need to qualify for permanent residence based upon an employment position. In a sense, there are four basic pathways to permanent residence based upon employment as a physician.

Pathway One

A highly attractive pathway to employment-based permanent residence is based upon the National Interest Waiver criteria. In this instance, an IMG has a streamlined, expedited pathway to permanent residence if it can be shown that his/her employment as a physician carries potential major benefits to areas of high national interest. If this can be established, the immigration filing is made directly to the Immigration and Naturalization Service, thereby skipping over entirely the filing process to the Department of Labor, as described below. Within a clinical setting, this National Interest Waiver strategy has been used over the years to facilitate the relocation of physicians to designated medically underserved areas.

The National Interest Waiver option was reinstated for physicians as a result of legislation passed into law in November 1999 and implemented by the Immigration and Naturalization Service in September 2000. At present, only primary care physicians working either in designated medically underserved areas or within the VA system may qualify for permanent resident status under this expedited approach of a National Interest Waiver. However, any physician seeking to gain his/her "green card" on the basis of this strategy needs first to have fulfilled a 5-year service commitment working specifically in a designated medically underserved area or within a VA facility.

Pathway Two

A second employment-based pathway to permanent residence involves a three-step process. The first and arguably most complex stage is the Labor Certification Application process. Conducted under the auspices of the US Department of Labor, this procedure establishes that employing a foreign national/IMG will not harm the US labor market, particularly by taking a job away from a fully qualified US worker. Therefore, acting under a complex recruitment/advertisement procedure, the employer needs to show that the IMG is not simply the most qualified applicant but is rather the only fully qualified candidate for the specific employment position.

After completing the Labor Certification Application process, the employer must submit an Immigrant Visa Petition to the Immigration and Naturalization Service

(INS), establishing the complete suitability of the IMG for the position. Upon approval of this petition, the IMG is able to actually apply for permanent residence either through an INS District Office (adjustment of status) or through a US Consular post (consular processing).

Note: An IMG needs to possess either an ECFMG certificate or an MD from an Liaison Committee for Medical Education (LCME)-accredited medical school (ie, generally Canadian or US). Also, an IMG cannot finalize the application for permanent residence status if he/she has an unfulfilled or unwaived J-1 2-year home residence obligation.

Pathway Three

A variant on the process above enables an employer to request a waiver of any further recruiting/advertising obligations. Such waivers are granted by the US Department of Labor when the employer has fully and in good faith recruited within the previous 6-month period, through which it legitimately came to the conclusion that there are no fully qualified US applicants for the open position.

Pathway Four

A final option to permanent residence is available to physicians of extraordinarily high professional capabilities, working either in clinical practice or in academic medicine. Such individuals may qualify for permanent residence under an expedited procedure established either for Aliens of Extraordinary Ability or Outstanding Professors or Researchers.

New Legal Developments

At present, the Conrad State 20 Waiver Program, as described above, is scheduled to sunset on June 1, 2002. This program empowers each state to recommend waivers for up to 20 IMGs per year, provided that they work in a designated medically underserved area for at least 3 years. At present, roughly 38 states have implemented their own waiver program. As of this writing, the Congress is starting consideration of extending and possibly even of expanding this program.

Effective February 27, 2002, the US Department of Agriculture announced a termination of its waiver program. As a result, the primary federal agency facilitating the relocation of IMGs to rural communities has stated its policy to withdraw from serving as an interested government agency for J-1 waiver purposes.

Many IMGs, particularly from third world countries, have traditionally processed for their visas through US Consulates in the neighboring countries of Canada or Mexico. A new law creates certain major new restrictions on visa processing in Canada or Mexico, although some concessions have been granted to physicians who intend to work in designated medically underserved communities. Furthermore, in the aftermath of September 11, all third world country foreign nationals, including IMGs, face increasing difficulty in obtaining visas through US Consulates in Canada or Mexico.

One new law cuts down considerably on instances in which the humanitarian benefits of a physician's services to a medically underserved area can be considered for the interim issuance of an employment authorization document.

Another recent law has also created major new bars to permanent residence for foreign nationals who have resided illegally within the United States for extended periods of time. This provision is certainly not targeted directly at physicians, but is rather an across-the-board provision intended to create a major new disincentive for violating US immigration laws.

The most wide-ranging legislative initiative of note involves the restoration of National Interest Waiver entitlement to physicians working within designated medically underserved areas and/or VA facilities. As noted above, permanent residence based upon the filing of a National Interest Waiver obligates the physician to fulfill a 5-year period of employment in a designated medically underserved area and/or a VA facility prior to gaining eligibility for permanent resident status. The purpose of this legislative initiative is to facilitate the relocation of physicians into employment positions that have traditionally been underserved by the domestic physician workforce.

Section IV.

Federal and National Programs and Activities

Licensure in the US Armed Forces

Department of the Air Force

Catherine E. Biersack, Colonel (S), USAF, MC
Chief, Clinical Quality Management Division
Air Force Medical Operations Agency/SGZC
Office of the Surgeon General
Washington DC

Sharon R. Ahrari, Lt Col, USAF, NC
Chief, Credentialing and Privileging Policy
Air Force Medical Operations Agency/SGZC
Office of the Surgeon General
Washington DC

The Clinical Quality Management Division of the Air Force Medical Operations Agency is responsible for oversight of clinical issues pertaining to quality improvement, licensure, credentialing and privileging, and risk management for the Air Force Surgeon General.

Air Force licensure policy is consistent with that of the Department of Defense (DOD). Air Force Medical Service physicians (military, civil service, contract personnel, and volunteers) must possess a current, valid, and unrestricted license from an official agency of a state; the District of Columbia; or a commonwealth, territory, or possession of the United States to provide health care independently within the scope of the license. Physicians must have a medical license that meets all clinical, professional, and administrative requirements of the issuing state and be no different than that of civilian counterparts.

Personnel accessed from professional training or who complete other training and require a license must obtain such license within 1 year of the date when all required didactic and clinical requirements are met, or within 1 year of completion of graduate year one. Physicians who do not yet meet licensure requirements may practice only under a written plan of supervision by a licensed, fully qualified, independently practicing, privileged provider of same or similar specialty. The Air Force requires physicians who choose to be licensed in a state that requires more than 1 year of graduate training to first obtain a license from a state that requires only 1 year of graduate training.

Department of the Army

Howard M. Kimes, Colonel, US Army
Director, Quality Management Directorate

Janet L. Wilson, Lieutenant Colonel, US Army
Chief, Regulatory Compliance
US Army Medical Command
Fort Sam Houston, Texas

The US Army Medical Command's Quality Management Directorate is responsible for developing policy and overseeing all facets of the Army Surgeon General's Quality Assurance Program, including quality improvement, credentials review and privileging, licensure, and risk management. The Directorate serves as the conduit for issues concerning clinical standards and accreditation by the Joint Commission for Accreditation of Healthcare Organizations for US Army Medicine Worldwide.

Department of Defense physicians (military and civilian, contractors and partners) must possess a current valid, unrestricted license from an official agency of the District of Columbia or a state, commonwealth, territory, or possession of the United States to provide health care independently within the scope of their licenses. Physicians in graduate medical education (GME) programs must possess a license within 1 year from the completion of their first year of GME training. An exception exists for individuals who complete their first year of GME in a state requiring 2 or more years of GME for licensure and who are assigned with that same state. These individuals must possess a license with in 1 year of completion of their second year of GME training.

Healthcare providers awaiting a required license work only under the supervision of a licensed provider.

Department of the Navy

Jan Chandler, Captain, Medical Corps, US Navy
Director, Clinical Operations
Bureau of Medicine and Surgery
Department of the Navy
Washington, DC

Georgi Irvine, Commander (Ret), Nurse Corps, US Navy
Head, Medical and Dental Staff Services
Naval Healthcare Support Office
Jacksonville, Florida

The Clinical Management and Plans Division within the Bureau of Medicine and Surgery, Department of the Navy (DON), is responsible for developing policy and directing the development and implementation of US Navy-wide quality management and professional affairs programs to improve the quality of patient care; reduce risks to our customers, guests, and staff; advance good stewardship; and maintain accreditation by the Joint Commission for Accreditation of Healthcare Organizations of all US Navy fixed medical treatment facilities.

Federal regulations require physicians and other health providers within the military health services system to possess a professional license or certification. The DON further requires the license to be current, valid, unrestricted, and one to which quality management data accrues. All DON physicians (military, civilian, civilian contract, and partnership), except interns, must possess a license from a recognized, official agency of a state; the District of Columbia; or a commonwealth, territory, or possession of the United States to provide health care services independently within the scope of their license. Licenses issued by authorities allowing reduced or no fees for military personnel must meet the same licensure criteria. Health care practitioners lacking required license or certification may work only under a plan of supervision with a licensed practitioner of the same or a similar professional discipline. This policy supports the US Navy's goal to ensure all practitioners are available for worldwide assignment and rapid deployment.

Federal Controlled Substances Registration

Office of Diversion Control
Drug Enforcement Administration
Washington, DC

Provisions of the Controlled Substances Act of 1970 (CSA) mandate that pharmaceuticals falling under its authority be maintained in a "closed system of distribution" that oversees all phases of manufacture, distribution, and dispensing. The Department of Justice, through the Drug Enforcement Administration (DEA), is entrusted with devising and administering a program that ensures the availability of controlled substances for the ultimate user, the patient, while preventing their diversion into illicit markets.

The backbone of the DEA's efforts is the controlled substances registration program. This program, through its implementing regulations, requires that any person desiring to manufacture, distribute, or dispense controlled substances must register with the DEA. After approval, each applicant is assigned a unique registration number, which must be used in every transaction involving controlled substances. Use of the DEA registration number, together with required records of transactions, allows tracking of controlled substances from the point of manufacture to the point at which they are dispensed to the patient.

As of April 3, 2002, there were 1,075,789 active DEA registrants. Medical practitioners account for 928,677 of those registrants, with an additional 65,000 new applications for registration received each year.

Applying for registration as a medical practitioner is a relatively simple process. A physician who seeks to become registered with the DEA must submit an application on DEA Form 224 together with the required fee to:

Drug Enforcement Administration
Registration Unit
PO Box 28083, Central Station
Washington, DC 20038-8083

The form can be obtained from the Registration Unit by calling 800 882-9539 or contacting any DEA field office with a registration assistant. Application forms are also available at the DEA Diversion Control Program Web site at www.DEAdiversion.usdoj.gov. The form can be completed online, printed, signed, and mailed to the above address.

Following initial processing by the Registration Unit, the application is referred to the appropriate DEA field office for a records check and verification with state licensing authorities that the practitioner is properly licensed and authorized by the state to handle controlled substances. Barring any problems, the registration is then approved and a certificate bearing the practitioner's DEA registration number is issued. This process normally takes from 4 to 6 weeks to complete. (Renewal applications generally are processed within 2 weeks.) The DEA certificate must be maintained at the registered location and must be kept available for official inspection.

Under special circumstances, applications may be faxed, but the completed forms cannot be returned for processing via facsimile. Completed applications must be mailed with the appropriate fee and an original signature. Completed application packages may be sent via overnight delivery, but the DEA will not incur the cost of any delivery service. Due to security requirements, all parcels received by the DEA are scanned in an off-site location prior to delivery. This requirement will add 1 day to the time it takes to receive packages. Non-US Postal Service deliveries should be addressed to:

Drug Enforcement Administration
attn: Registration Unit, ODRR
2401 Jefferson Davis Highway
Alexandria, VA 22301

The DEA also registers mid-level practitioners (MLPs) who have been authorized by the appropriate state licensing agency to handle controlled substances. Currently over 71,000 MLPs, including nurse practitioners, certified nurse-midwives, physician assistants, and optometrists, are registered with the DEA. MLPs apply for registration on the same application forms as other practitioners. MLP registration numbers begin with the letter "M" rather than the letters "A" or "B," which are issued to other practitioners.

The fee for both new and renewal applications for all practitioners is $210 for a 3-year period. The exemption from payment of the application fee is limited to federal, state, or local government-operated hospitals or institutions.

A practitioner's registration must be renewed every 3 years. Each practitioner is issued a renewal application, DEA Form 224a, approximately 45 days before the expiration date of his or her registration. Registrants who do not receive the form can contact any local DEA office with a registration assistant. DEA registrations are issued for controlled substances activities at specific locations. If a physician has more than one office at which controlled substances will be administered and/or dispensed, a separate registration must be obtained for each location. However, this requirement applies only to those locations away from the principal location at which controlled substances will be administered or dispensed. If the activities at secondary locations are restricted to prescribing only within the same state, then separate registration is not required.

When dealing with the DEA on registration issues, practitioners should be aware of the following:

1. When filing a new or renewal application, or requesting modification of a registration, file early; DEA's registration program receives over 400,000 filings per year.

2. One of the primary criteria for issuing a DEA registration is that the applicant be authorized by the state in which he or she will practice. Make sure that all necessary applications, etc, for state licensing have been taken care of before filing your application for DEA registration. The same applies for registrants relocating from one state to another.

3. Keep track of your registration expiration date. Between 20,000 and 30,000 renewal notices are mailed to registrants each month. There is no guarantee that all of them will be received by the registrants. If a registration does expire, that registration cannot be used for any purpose, and the registrant is no longer authorized to handle controlled substances. Until the registration is renewed and a new certificate of registration is issued, use of the registration is a violation of the law.

4. As noted earlier, DEA registrations are issued for controlled substances activities at a specific location. Therefore, the Registration Unit or appropriate DEA field office must be notified in advance of any change of address. Further, the registration address cannot be a post office box but the actual location at which controlled substances activities take place. If there are problems with postal delivery or the address that should be used, contact the Registration Unit or local DEA office before filing.

5. The Registration Unit can be contacted toll-free at

   800 882-9539

   Whenever contacting the DEA regarding an existing registration, reference the DEA registration number. Further, if the matter is considered important, conduct it in writing. During busy periods, the Registration Unit receives thousands of calls each week; a mental note is easier to lose than a letter.

The DEA's registration program plays an extremely important role in efforts to control the diversion of legitimately produced controlled substances to the illicit market. The program has grown in complexity with the addition of new substances, such as anabolic steroids, and a new category of registration—mid-level practitioners—for advanced practice nurses, certified nurse midwives, physician assistants, and others. The continued success of the program is the result of the combined efforts and understanding of health care professionals, industry, and the DEA.

The answer to many registration questions and locations of DEA field offices and registration assistants are listed on the Diversion Control Program Web site, available at

www.DEAdiversion.usdoj.gov.

National Practitioner Data Bank and Healthcare Integrity and Protection Data Bank

These two federal programs collect specific data nationwide about health care practitioners, providers, and suppliers.

The National Practitioner Data Bank (NPDB) collects and releases information on physicians' medical malpractice payments, adverse licensure actions, adverse clinical privilege actions, adverse professional society membership actions, and exclusions from participation in Medicare and Medicaid. The NPDB is a flagging system that facilitates a comprehensive review of actions affecting health care practitioners' professional credentials. Hospitals, managed care organizations, other authorized health care entities, professional societies, and state licensing boards use NPDB information, in conjunction with other sources, when granting clinical privileges or when making employment, affiliation, or licensure decisions. Hospitals, professional societies, and other health care organizations are also required to report certain data to the NPDB. Malpractice insurers must report all payments made for individual practitioners.

The Healthcare Integrity and Protection Data Bank (HIPDB) collects and releases information on health care practitioners, providers, and suppliers' licensure and certification actions, exclusions from participation in federal and state health care programs, criminal convictions and civil judgments related to health care, and other adjudicated actions or decisions. The HIPDB is an alert or flagging system that assists federal and state agencies, state licensing boards, and health plans in conducting extensive, independent investigations of the qualifications of health care practitioners, providers, or suppliers whom they seek to license, hire, or credential, or with whom they seek to contract or affiliate. Health plans and federal and state government agencies are required to report certain data to the HIPDB.

Both Data Banks are operated under the direct supervision of the Division of Practitioner Data Banks, Bureau of Health Professions, Health Resources and Services Administration, US Department of Health and Human Services (HHS), although the HHS Office of the Inspector General has statutory responsibility for the HIPDB. The NPDB began collecting and disseminating information in 1990. The HIPDB began collecting information in 1999 and disseminating it in 2000.

Data Availability and Confidentiality

Information reported to the NPDB and HIPDB is considered confidential. NPDB information is available only to state licensing boards; hospitals and other health care entities, including professional societies; and others as specified in the law. HIPDB information is available only to health plans and federal and state government agencies. Information that identifies individuals is not available to the general public. Statistical information is made available to the public.

Healthcare practitioners, providers, and suppliers are allowed to query their own records in the NPDB and HIPDB at any time. All self-query requests are automatically sent to both Data Banks, and a fee of $10 is assessed by each Data Bank. A self-query may not be sent to only one Data Bank. Subjects of a report in either Data Bank receive with their self-query responses a list of all parties to whom the report has been disclosed.

Reporting, Statements, and Disputing Reports

NPDB and HIPDB reporting and querying are done through an Internet-based system, the Integrated Querying and Reporting Service (IQRS). NPDB and HIPDB reporting are combined into one system, with a set of rules determining how reports are accepted into each Data Bank. Based upon the information reported, the IQRS routes reporting transactions to the appropriate Data Bank(s).

After processing a report from a reporting entity, the NPDB and HIPDB sends a notice to the entity and to the individual or organizations ("subjects") mentioned in the report. If there are errors, subjects must ask the reporting entity to correct the information. Both Data Banks are prohibited from modifying information submitted in reports except through a "Secretarial Review" process established to resolve disputed reports not corrected by the reporting entities.

Subjects of a NPDB or HIPDB report may add a statement to the report, dispute either the factual accuracy of the information in a report or whether the report was submitted in accordance with NPDB or HIPDB reporting requirements, or both. If the reporting entity does not make a correction satisfactory to the subject of a report, the subject may request "Secretarial Review." The HHS will then review whether the report was legally field and accurate.

Responsibilities of State Boards

State licensing boards must report to the NPDB certain adverse licensure actions related to professional competence or professional conduct and any changes to such actions. These actions include revocation, suspension, censure, reprimand, probation, and surrender. Boards must also report revisions to adverse licensure actions. State boards must report to the HIPDB final adverse actions taken against health care practitioners, providers, or suppliers.

Available Materials

Materials available from the Data Banks include the National Practitioner Data Bank *Guidebook*; Healthcare Integrity and Protection Data Bank *Guidebook*; fact sheets on various topics; and self-query materials. All the materials are available on the Internet at www.npdb-hipdb.com.

National Practitioner Data Bank and
Healthcare Integrity and Protection Data Bank
PO Box 10832
Chantilly, VA 20151
800 767-6732
www.npdb-hipdb.com

Other Organizations and Programs

American Board of Medical Specialties

The American Board of Medical Specialties (ABMS) is a nonprofit organization of 24 approved medical specialty boards. These 24 boards (listed below) have been approved by the ABMS and the AMA Council on Medical Education (AMA CME) through the Liaison Committee for Specialty Boards (LCSB), with ultimate approval of the application by the membership of the ABMS and the AMA CME.

American Board of:

- Allergy and Immunology
- Anesthesiology
- Colon and Rectal Surgery
- Dermatology
- Emergency Medicine
- Family Practice
- Internal Medicine
- Medical Genetics
- Neurological Surgery
- Nuclear Medicine
- Obstetrics and Gynecology
- Ophthalmology
- Orthopaedic Surgery
- Otolaryngology
- Pathology
- Pediatrics
- Physical Medicine and Rehabilitation
- Plastic Surgery
- Preventive Medicine
- Psychiatry and Neurology
- Radiology
- Surgery
- Thoracic Surgery
- Urology

Mission of the ABMS

The mission of the ABMS is to maintain and improve the quality of medical care by helping its member boards develop and use professional and educational standards for the evaluation and certification of physician specialists. The certification of physicians provides assurance to the public that a physician specialist certified by an ABMS member board has successfully completed an approved educational program and an evaluation process that assesses the knowledge, skills, and experience required to provide quality patient care in that specialty. Medical specialty board certification is an additional process to receiving a medical degree, completing residency training, and receiving a license to practice medicine.

In collaboration with the other organizations and agencies concerned, the approved medical specialty boards assist in improving the quality of medical education by elevating the standards of graduate medical education and approving facilities for specialty training.

The actual accreditation review for the approval of residency programs in each specialty is conducted by a Residency Review Committee on which the respective specialty board has equal representation with the AMA Council on Medical Education and, in some cases, with a related specialty society.

Maintenance of Certification

A major focus of the 24 medical specialty member boards of the ABMS is initial certification, a rigorous process that evaluates the training, qualifications, and competence of physician specialists at the outset of their careers. In addition to initial certification, ABMS and its member boards are committed to ensuring the ongoing competence of board-certified physician specialists. Currently, this is done through "recertification programs" in which doctors are evaluated every 7-10 years, primarily by a written examination. The ABMS member boards have determined that this system needs to be expanded to more fully assess the continuing competence of physicians.

To better evaluate the competence of physician specialists throughout their careers, ABMS Member Boards are in the process of moving from "recertification" to a more comprehensive plan called "maintenance of certification." Maintenance of Cetification© is an in-depth program that will be continuous and relevant to practice. A key component of the emerging Maintenance of Certification program is the evaluation of physician practice performance including six core competencies (patient care, medical knowledge, interpersonal and communication skills, professionalism, practice-based learning and improvement, and systems-based practice).

Since the ABMS Maintenance of Certification program will involve most US physicians and will include assessment of physician practice performance and quality improvement initiatives in the six core competencies, it should eventually lead to enhanced quality of care provided by physicians and better patient health care outcomes.

Contact Information

For more information about the ABMS, its member boards, and the process of developing and using standards for the evaluation and certification of physician specialists, contact:

American Board of Medical Specialties
1007 Church St/Ste 404
Evanston, IL 60201-5913
847 491-9091
847 328-3596 Fax
www.abms.org

Medical Specialty Board Certification and its Relationship to Licensure

Stephen H. Miller, MD, MPH
Executive Vice President
American Board of Medical Specialties
Evanston, Illinois

Arthur Osteen, PhD
Former Director
Department of PRA, Policy and Liaison Activities
American Medical Association
Chicago, Illinois

From its inception, medical specialty certification in the United States has been a voluntary process. Since the establishment of the first nationally recognized medical specialty board in 1917, some physicians have elected to seek formal recognition of their qualifications in their chosen specialty fields by presenting themselves for examination before specialty boards composed of their professional peers. The definitions of each of the specialties and of the educational and other requirements leading to eligibility for board certification have been developed by consensus within the medical profession. This process of certification of a medical specialist has remained separate and distinct from licensure by civil authorities of professionals qualified to practice medicine within their jurisdictions.

The American Board of Medical Specialties (ABMS) is the umbrella organization for the 24 medical specialty boards authorized and recognized to certify physician specialists in the United States. The 24 boards have been approved by the ABMS and the AMA Council on Medical Education (AMA CME) through the Liaison Committee for Specialty Boards (LCSB), with ultimate approval of the application by the membership of the ABMS and the AMA CME.

The primary function of the ABMS is to maintain and improve the quality of medical care by assisting the member boards in their efforts to develop and use standards for the evaluation and certification of physician specialists. The intent of the certification process is to improve the quality of patient care by providing assurance to the public that a certified physician specialist has successfully completed an approved educational program and an evaluation, including an examination process designed to assess the knowledge, skills, and experience necessary for the provision of quality patient care in that specialty.

ABMS Statement on "Relationship Between Specialty Board Certification and Medical Licensure"

The ABMS encourages its member boards to require unlimited medical licensure as a prerequisite for certification and maintenance of such licensure for recertification. This is one of several criteria the boards may use in satisfying themselves as to the moral character and legal standing of candidates in their respective states. A number of state licensing boards now accept certification by a specialty board in lieu of their own requirements for licensure.

Although the ABMS recognizes the right of each state to establish its own regulations, ABMS discourages the substitution of certification for licensure requirements because it has led in some cases to licensure by specialty. The ABMS opposes licensure by specialty for the following reasons:

1. It is convinced that every specialist should maintain basic knowledge and skill in the broad aspects of medical care.

2. The boundaries between specialties are often hazy and overlapping. State governments should not define such boundaries lest transgressions be punishable under the law. ABMS believes that practice restrictions should be determined only by the judgment of individual physicians, the medical staffs of hospitals, or the customs of the community in which the doctor practices.

3. Licensure by specialty will impose serious handicaps on physicians who seek interstate endorsement of licenses so obtained. Very few state licensing boards will endorse licenses obtained by specialty certification.

4. Requiring a physician to limit his or her practice to a specialty could increase the cost of medical care as it might entail needless consultations with unnecessary repetition of tests with concomitant increases in patients' bills.

Furthermore, the laws of many states either permit or require licensing boards to establish rules and regulations mandating continuing medical education (CME) for reregistration of medical licenses. Some state boards will accept specialty board recertification as satisfying their CME requirements.

Although the ABMS recognizes the right of each state to establish its own regulations, it discourages the acceptance of recertification in lieu of the state's reregistration requirements for the following reasons:

1. There is danger that this could encourage a trend toward licensure by specialty.

2. As recertification is private and voluntary, it is undesirable to adopt this as a substitute for the public and legal requirements of licensing boards.

Approved by the ABMS Assembly, January 28, 1977; reaffirmed on March 20, 1997.

Definition of "Board Eligible"

"Board eligible" is a term frequently used to describe a physician who has completed a period of specialty education but has not been specialty board certified. Usually the term is understood to mean that the physician has completed the years of graduate medical education required for certification but has not taken the specialty board examination.

Official ABMS policy states that the term "board eligible" should not be used. Instead, physicians and medical organizations should state exactly what a physician's circumstances are in regard to certification. For example, physicians planning to seek or seeking board certification might state that they have completed the years of residency required for admission to the examination, have been admitted to the examination, or have passed the examination and will be provided with a certificate. Physicians who do not plan to seek board certification should specifically state their qualifications for practice, including any special training or honors.

AMA Policy Regarding Specialty Board Certification and Licensure

AMA policy, like that of the ABMS, opposes licensure by specialty. The earliest statement of this policy comes in a report of the AMA Council on Medical Education (CME):

> "Experience with licensure by specialty is too limited to determine what the long-range effects will be in the provision of timely, safe, and comprehensive medical care. However, the AMA does not consider licensure by specialty to be desirable even in unusual cases."

This position was reaffirmed by a report of the Council on Long Range Planning and Development in 1990. Discussions in CME meetings indicate support for the position that all physicians, regardless of specialty, should have knowledge of general medicine, that is, they should be able to identify illnesses and disorders and refer patients to other physicians if needed. Licensure based on specialty education and specialty examinations would be insufficient to ensure that physicians have a broad base of general medical knowledge.

The AMA has also adopted a policy that hospitals and managed care organizations should be able to appoint to staff physicians who do not have specialty board certificates. The most recent statement of this policy is from AMA CME Report 5, adopted in 1996:

> "[It is recommended that] the AMA reaffirm policy that decisions regarding staff appointment should be based upon the training, experience, and demonstrated competence of candidates and not exclusively upon the presence or absence of board certification; and that third party payers not exclude non-board certified physicians as a class from participation in their programs, without regard to individual training, experience, and current competence."

The AMA has communicated the policy to hospitals and to managed care organizations, many of which have physicians on staff who do not have specialty board certificates.

The AMA recognizes the importance of specialty board certification and supports the certification process. The AMA, for instance, is a member of the Liaison Committee on Specialty Boards, which has established procedures for the recognition of new boards that become members of the ABMS. The AMA also recognizes that there are competent physicians who do not have board certificates.

Accreditation Council for Graduate Medical Education

The Accreditation Council for Graduate Medical Education (ACGME) is an accrediting agency composed of directors nominated by five national associations interested in graduate medical education: the American Board of Medical Specialties, American Hospital Association, American Medical Association, Association of American Medical Colleges, and Council of Medical Specialty Societies.

The federal government names a representative to serve in a nonvoting capacity, and the ACGME chooses three public directors. There is also a resident director appointed by the Resident Physicians Section of the AMA, with the advice of other national organizations that represent residents, and the chair of the Residency Review Committee Council sits as a voting director.

A Residency Review Committee (RRC) consists of representatives appointed by the AMA, the appropriate specialty board, and, in some cases, a national specialty organization. The Transitional Year Review Committee is composed of nine members who are appointed by the chair of the ACGME in conjunction with the Executive Committee. The term "review committee" is used to denote a Residency Review Committee and the Transitional Year Review Committee.

GME programs are accredited either by the ACGME upon the recommendation of an appropriate review committee, or by the review committee itself, if accreditation authority has been delegated by the ACGME. Accreditation of a residency program indicates that it is judged to be in substantial compliance with the *Essentials of Accredited Residencies in Graduate Medical Education* (*Essentials*), which includes the Institutional Requirements and the relevant Program Requirements. The jurisdiction of the ACGME is limited to programs in the United States, its territories, and its possessions.

A list of programs accredited by the ACGME, including detailed information about each program, is published annually by the AMA in the *Graduate Medical Education Directory*. The most current listing can also be found on the ACGME Web site at www.acgme.org. With the exception of that information, the contents of program files are confidential, as are all other documents regarding a program used by a review committee.

ACGME General Competencies

In 1999, responding in part to growing criticism that residents/fellows were not adequately prepared to practice in the rapidly changing health care environment, the ACGME endorsed General Competencies in the six areas below. ACGME Program Requirements state that GME programs must define the specific knowledge, skills, and attitudes required and provide educational experiences as needed in order for their residents/fellows to demonstrate these competencies to the level expected of a new practitioner.

Patient Care that is compassionate, appropriate, and effective for the treatment of health problems and the promotion of health

Medical Knowledge about established and evolving biomedical, clinical, and cognate (eg, epidemiological and social-behavioral) sciences and the application of this knowledge to patient care

Practice-Based Learning and Improvement that involves investigation and evaluation of their own patient care, appraisal and assimilation of scientific evidence, and improvements in patient care

Interpersonal and Communication Skills that result in effective information exchange and teaming with patients, their families, and other health professionals

Professionalism, as manifested through a commitment to carrying out professional responsibilities, adherence to ethical principles, and sensitivity to a diverse patient population

Systems-Based Practice, as manifested by actions that demonstrate an awareness of and responsiveness to the larger context and system of health care and the ability to effectively call on system resources to provide care of optimal value.

Contact Information

Accreditation Council for Graduate Medical Education
515 N State St, 20th Fl
Chicago, IL 60610
312 464-4920   312 464-4098 Fax
www.acgme.org

American Medical Association Survey and Data Resources

The AMA Division of Survey and Data Resources is dedicated to effectively collecting, analyzing and managing physician data.

The chief function of the division is maintaining the AMA Physician Masterfile, a database of current and historical data on over 800,000 physicians in the US, both AMA members and nonmembers. This figure includes approximately 190,000 graduates of foreign medical schools who reside in the United States and who have met the educational and credentialing requirements necessary for recognition and approximately 45,000 doctors of osteopathy. Physician records are never removed from the AMA Physician Masterfile. Records of deceased physicians are shared with other organizations and are used to identify individuals who fraudulently attempt to assume the credentials of deceased physicians.

Survey and Data Resources comprises three departments:

- Data Collection
- Physician Practice and Communications Information
- Physician Data and Internet Services.

These departments are essential in maintaining the Masterfile as the most comprehensive and accurate source of physician data.

Data Collection

The Department of Data Collection is where each individual AMA Physician Masterfile record is first established. This occurs when individuals enter medical schools accredited by the Liaison Committee on Medical Education (LCME) in the US or Canada. In the case of international medical graduates, a record is established upon entry into residency programs accredited by the Accreditation Council for Graduate Medical Education (ACGME). Background information on these individuals is also verified with the Educational Commission for Foreign Medical Graduates (ECFMG). Doctors of osteopathy are

added to the Masterfile through AMA annual surveys, membership solicitation, or through the processing of new licensure data as reported by state licensing boards.

As new records are created, Data Collection assigns a record identifier called the Medical Education (ME) number. This number remains the same throughout a physician's medical career.

Each record within the Masterfile contains information which is "primary source"-reported from over 2,100 different medical organizations, institutions, and government agencies. This means that student information is received from medical schools, residency program directors, and so on.

A major function of the Data Collection department is the processing of resident information collected via the National GME Census. This survey, historically administered by the Data Collection department, is now conducted online in a joint effort with the Association of American Medical Colleges. Each year approximately 8,000 ACGME-accredited and ABMS Board-approved GME programs are surveyed in addition to 1,600 teaching institutions. The reported residency information is internally validated before it is incorporated into a physician's record. The survey also includes questions on GME program characteristics, such as clinical and research facilities and the learning environment, which are used to update FREIDA Online (www.ama-assn.org/go/freida) and the *Graduate Medical Education Directory*, produced by the Medical Education group.

Data Collection is also responsible for processing all active and historical licensure information on US physicians. The department receives and processes approximately 11 million updates annually from the 67 medical and osteopathic jurisdictions that license physicians. Additionally, the department performs quarterly updates to board certification information for over 700,000 physician records, as reported by the American Board of Medical Specialties, and monthly updates to controlled substance registration information for over 30,000 physician records, as reported by the US Department of Justice Drug Enforcement Administration.

A system called CAM (Computer Aided Matching) is used to match the ME number to other numerically based information, such as state license or board certification number. This system helps in processing the 14 million records received each year by the department.

Physician Practice and Communications Information

Once physicians complete residency and/or fellowship training, the Department of Physician Practice and Communications Information begins to track them through periodic surveys.

The Census of Physicians, for example, collects information on a physician's professional medical activities, preferred address, principal hospital and group affiliation, present employment, and practice specialties, among other data. The information is used to communicate with physicians, segment physician markets, draw samples for health-related research, and track professional trends.

The Department of Physician Practice and Communications Information also surveys medical group practices in order to maintain the Group Practice Database, which contains information on over 20,000 group practices. These data are used for a service available through the AMA Web site, Group Select, membership development, and marketing products and services.

Another function of this unit is to maintain address information for the Physician Masterfile. Each year, approximately 250,000 physician addresses are updated. To ensure high-quality and deliverable addresses, the AMA subscribes to the USPS Address Correction System (ACS) and maintains biannual certification by the National Change of Address Services (NCOA).

Finally, the department is responsible for producing an annual publication of summary statistics on the population of physicians, *Physician Characteristics and Distribution in the US.*

Physician Data and Internet Services

The Department of Physician Data and Internet Services manages the AMA's data procurement activities. This department is responsible for building and maintaining data exchange relationships, so that the AMA continues to obtain and manage valuable physician information. The unit serves as a liaison with outside organizations from which it receives data (eg, licensing boards, certifying agencies, and professional associations).

A major function of the Department of Physician Data and Internet Services is to collect physician licensure and disciplinary action data. For many years the AMA has collected active and historical licensure data from the 67 jurisdictions that license physicians. In 1997, the AMA expanded its procurement activities to include physician disciplinary data. To date, 66 of the 67 US licensing jurisdictions, the US Department of Health and Human Services, and the US Department of Justice Drug Enforcement Administration have reported physician disciplinary data spanning as far back as a decade. The AMA has received nationwide recognition as the only entity that maintains a complete history of physician-specific licensure activity across allopathic and osteopathic licensing authorities.

The department is also responsible for reporting critical physician credential information to hospitals, managed care organizations, medical schools, state licensing boards, and other organizations concerned with verifying physicians' credentials. The AMA Physician Profile is a printout containing such information as physician name, professional mailing address, date and place of birth, medical education, residency training, state licensure, and specialty board certification. Through the use of the Physician Profile, organizations can verify credentials, detect impostors or dishonest physicians, and identify those who have been disciplined by a licensing board or federal agency. The Physician Profile helps strengthen the medical profession by ensuring that only the most qualified physicians are allowed to care for the public's health. Over 350,000 Physician Profiles are generated annually.

Physician Data and Internet Services also manages an internal application for the maintenance of mailing lists or contact management information supporting key Association activities. This application currently contains over 100 different list directories, including AMA board, council, committee, and advisory group members; and executive staff of state, county, and national medical specialty societies. It supports Association mailings related to special activities or events and is also used to update the Federation and Pictorial Directories published on the AMA Web site. Through this application, over 120,000 mailing labels are generated each year.

The AMA Physician Masterfile is a data source not only for internal use but also for use by other professional medical organizations, universities and medical schools, research institutions, governmental agencies, and other related groups. Providing services to agencies and organizations concerned with verifying physicians' credentials is essential to the AMA's mission. It is one of the many ways in which the Association works to strengthen the medical profession and ensure quality health care for the American public.

Contact Information

Division of Survey and Data Resources
Kevin Kenward, PhD, Director
312 464-4919

Department of Data Collection
Pam Rosinski, Director
312 464-4050

Department of Physician Practice
and Communications Information
Penny Havlicek, PhD, Director
312 464-5318

Department of Physician Data and Internet Services
Monica Quiroz, Director
312 464-4153

E-mail: PhysData@ama-assn.org
www.ama-assn.org/ama/pub/category/2670.html

American Medical Association Continuing Medical Education

Advances in biomedical science and changes in the other facets of the US health care delivery environment engage physicians in a continuous process of professional development. To ensure that they provide patients with the most current and appropriate treatment, services, and information, physicians keep learning through participation in a wide array of conferences and other teaching experiences, as well as through independent study of published materials. The American Medical Association (AMA) supports these physician efforts by:

- administering the only non-specialty-specific credit system that recognizes physician completion of continuing medical education (CME) activities;
- providing online information about accredited CME activities through the CME Locator;
- offering CME publications and programs (both conferences and enduring materials, such as monographs and course materials); and
- exploring new learning modalities appropriate for physician professional development and investigating international opportunities for reciprocal CME relationships.

The AMA Physician's Recognition Award

In 1968, the AMA House of Delegates established the AMA Physician's Recognition Award (PRA) to both encourage physicians to participate in CME and acknowledge when individual physicians complete CME activities. Approximately 20,000 physicians apply for the PRA each year, with 60,000 holding current AMA PRA certificates. Activities that meet education standards established by the AMA can be designated "AMA PRA category 1" by educational institutions accredited to provide CME to US physicians. These typically include state medical societies, medical specialty societies, medical schools, and hospitals. Other activities, usually independent or physician directed learning, may be reported for Category 2.

AMA PRA certificates are awarded in lengths of 1, 2, or 3 years, with the following requirements:

1-year certificate – 50 hours
- 20 hours category 1
- 30 hours category 1 or 2

2-year certificate – 100 hours
- 40 hours category 1
- 60 hours category 1 or 2

3-year certificate – 150 hours
- 60 hours category 1
- 90 hours category 1 or 2

Through reciprocity arrangements, the AMA will also award the PRA certificate if the CME requirements of the following organizations are met:

- American Academy of Dermatology
- American Academy of Family Physicians
- American Academy of Ophthalmology
- American Academy of Otolaryngology - Head and Neck Surgery
- American Academy of Pediatrics
- American College of Obstetricians and Gynecologists
- American College of Emergency Physicians
- American College of Preventive Medicine
- American Psychiatric Association
- American Society of Anesthesiologists
- American Society of Clinical Pathologists/ College of American Pathologists
- American Society of Plastic Surgeons
- American Urological Association Education and Research
- California Medical Association
- Medical Society of New Jersey
- Medical Society of Virginia
- National Medical Association

In addition, the following states accept the PRA certificate as evidence that physicians have met the CME requirements for license reregistration:

- Alabama
- Alaska
- California
- Delaware
- Hawaii
- Illinois
- Iowa
- Kansas
- Maine
- Michigan
- Minnesota
- Mississippi
- New Hampshire
- New Mexico
- North Dakota
- Ohio
- Oklahoma
- Washington
- West Virginia

The AMA sends PRA application forms to physicians who have had a valid PRA certificate within the past 3 years, physicians whose current certificate is expiring within 3 months, and resident physicians who have completed at least 3 years of graduate medical education. The AMA PRA application form and the PRA Information Booklet, available in physician and provider versions, are also available online at www.ama-assn.org/go/pra or by contacting:

Department of Accreditation and Certification Activities
Continuing Physician Professional Development
American Medical Association
515 N State St
Chicago, IL 60610
312 464-4941
312 464-4567 Fax
E-mail: pra@ama-assn.org

For bulk orders of the AMA Physician's Recognition Award Booklet, available in physician and provider versions, please contact the AMA Order Department at 800 621-8335.

Online Information About Accredited CME Activities

The AMA Online CME Locator, available at www.ama-assn.org/go/cme/locator, is a database of more than 2,000 category 1 activities for the AMA PRA. All listed sponsors are accredited by the Accreditation Council for Continuing Medical Education.

AMA CME Programs

Enduring (Self-Assessment) CME Programs

The AMA Healthcare Education Products Group offers a number of enduring CME programs that provide physician self-assessment. These programs offer quality CME in a convenient format that permits learners to work at their own pace and at a time that fits a busy clinical schedule. Available in print, CD-ROM, and Internet formats, these enduring CME programs are dedicated to improving the effectiveness and scope of CME programs by exploring new formats and delivery approaches that tap into the latest clinical information and that meet the AMA's rigorous CME standards.

Monographs/Internet Programs

The AMA Division of Healthcare Education Products and Standards produces and distributes both printed self-study monographs and Internet/CD-ROM programs, which are developed in cooperation with medical specialty societies and recognized medical experts and funded with educational grant support from industry. These programs are intended for primary care physicians and other interested medical specialists. Programs are available in the following areas:

Respiratory Disorders
- Managing Asthma Today (I): Integrating New Concepts
  2 hours, Print and Internet
- Managing Asthma Today (II): Common Comorbidities and Select Patient Populations
  2 hours, Print and Internet

Viral STDs

- Genital Herpes: A Clinician's Guide to Diagnosis and Treatment
  3 hours, Print

Neurological Conditions

- Managing Migraine Today (I): Diagnosis and Principles of Care
  2 hours, Print and Internet

- Managing Migraine Today (II): Pharmacologic & Nonpharmacologic Treatment
  2 hours, Print and Internet

Medical Genetics

- Identifying and Managing Hereditary Risk for Breast and Ovarian Cancer
  3 hours, Print

- Identifying and Managing Risk for Hereditary Nonpolyposis Colorectal Cancer and Endometrial Cancer (HNPCC)
  3 hours, Print

Gastrointestinal Disease

- New Considerations in the Diagnosis and Management of Gastroesophageal Reflux Disease (GERD)
  3 hours, Print

Endocrine and Metabolic Disorders

- Managing Diabetes (I): Understanding Type 2 Diabetes
  3 hours, Print/pdf

- Managing Diabetes (II): Treatment Issues in Type 2 Diabetes
  3 hours, Print/pdf

- Managing Diabetes (III): Complications of Diabetes
  3 hours, Print/pdf

- Diabetes Case Study #1: Young Hispanic Woman
  1 hour, Internet

- Diabetes Case Study #2: Middle-Aged Afro-American Male
  1 hour, Internet

- Diabetes Case Study #3: 53-Year Old Hispanic Man
  1 hour, Internet

Osteoporosis

- Managing Osteoporosis (I): Detection and Clinical Issues in Testing
  3 hours, Print and Internet

- Managing Osteoporosis (II): Glucocorticoid-Induced Osteoporosis
  3 hours, Print and Internet

- Managing Osteoporosis (III): Prevention and Treatment of Postmenopausal Osteoporosis
  3 hours, Print and Internet

- Managing Osteoporosis (IV): Update in Patient Management
  3 hours, Print and Internet

- 4-part series also available in CD ROM

Disorders of the Immune System, Connective Tissue, and Joints

- Managing Osteoarthritis: Diagnosis and Principles of Care
  2 hours, Print and Internet

Journal CME

Since 1997, the AMA has designated selected articles in the *Journal of the American Medical Association (JAMA)* Reader's Choice and the AMA Archives journals (listed below) for AMA PRA category 1 credit.

- *Archives of Dermatology*
- *Archives of Facial Plastic Surgery*
- *Archives of General Psychiatry*
- *Archives of Internal Medicine*
- *Archives of Neurology*
- *Archives of Ophthalmology*
- *Archives of Otolaryngology - Head & Neck Surgery*
- *Archives of Pediatrics & Adolescent Medicine*
- *Archives of Surgery*

AMA-sponsored Conferences and Live Events

As an ACCME-accredited provider, the AMA sponsors multiple conferences and live events designated for AMA PRA category 1 credit. Physicians receive education on topics of interest to all disciplines and specialties. In recent years AMA-sponsored conferences and live events have included the AMA National Leadership Conference, the 11th World Conference on Tobacco OR Health, and the AMA-Internet Health Road Show.

International CME

The International Conference Recognition Program started in 1990 by an act of the American Medical Association (AMA) House of Delegates. The AMA recognized that international congresses present opportunities for physicians to participate in quality educational programs and provide opportunities for US physicians to collaborate with colleagues overseas. The AMA recognizes a handful of events each year and provides American physicians with an opportunity to earn AMA PRA category 1 credit at these approved events. For more information, contact Julie Johnston at 312 464-5196.

Contact Information

For more information on AMA CME programs and activities, visit www.ama-assn.org/go/cme or contact:

Multimedia CME	312 464-5990
AMA CME credits/courses	312 464-4637
Physician's Recognition Award	312 464-4672
International CME	312 464-5196

For general information, contact:

Continuing Physician Professional Development
American Medical Association
515 N State St
Chicago, IL 60610
312 464-4671
312 464-5830 Fax
E-mail: cppd@ama-assn.org

American Medical Association Project USA

Now more than a quarter of a century old, Project USA is the American Medical Association's program that recruits physicians for short-term service in rural areas. Funded by the US Public Health Service, Project USA is a coordinated effort involving the AMA and the Indian Health Service. The purpose of the program is to provide temporary short-term replacements for Public Health Service physicians, enabling them to take vacations or fulfill continuing education requirements.

Primary care physicians with a full and unrestricted license to practice medicine are being sought to participate in Project USA. Openings are available year round for 2 to 4 weeks or longer. These locum tenens positions provide a weekly salary, malpractice insurance coverage, and round-trip coach airfare; housing accommodations are also available.

Project USA volunteers may be part of a health care team that includes dentists, nurses, and other health personnel while serving at a three- or four-doctor Indian Health Service hospital, or may work in a solo-practice setting.

The Need for Project USA

Medically underserved rural areas are in need of the continuing medical services that physicians can provide. Physicians who volunteer for Project USA have an opportunity to become exposed to totally different cultures and to find new perspectives and insights, both medical and social. They also enjoy the satisfaction that comes from responding to a need for their professional services and the appreciation of rural people for their contributions to the health care of their community.

Contact Information

John Naughton, Project Director
Project USA, American Medical Association
515 N State St
Chicago, IL 60610
312 464-4702
800 388-4702
312 464-4184 Fax
E-mail: john_naughton@ama-assn.org
www.ama-assn.org/go/projectusa

Joint Commission on Accreditation of Healthcare Organizations

An independent, nonprofit organization, the Joint Commission on Accreditation of Healthcare Organizations (JCAHO), or Joint Commission, evaluates and accredits almost 18,000 health care organizations and programs in the United States and other countries. Accreditation by the Joint Commission is nationally recognized as a symbol of quality indicating that an organization meets state-of-the-art performance standards.

Joint Commission staff work with health care experts, providers, researchers, purchasers, and consumers around the world to develop optimally achievable performance standards, all with a single focus—to improve the safety and quality of patient care.

To earn and maintain accreditation, organizations must undergo an on-site survey by a team of Joint Commission surveyors at least every 3 years (laboratories are surveyed every 2 years). The Joint Commission employs more than 400 experienced physicians, nurses, health care administrators, medical technologists, psychologists, pharmacists, and other medical professionals to conduct these surveys.

Accreditation Programs

The Joint Commission operates the eight accreditation programs, listed below, that serve various types of health care organizations:

- *Assisted Living Accreditation Program*
- *Hospital Accreditation Program*
- *Home Care Accreditation Program*
- *Ambulatory Care Accreditation Program*
- *Laboratory Accreditation Program*
- *Long Term Care Accreditation Program*
- *Behavioral Health Care Accreditation Program*
- *Network Accreditation Program*

Benefits of Accreditation

Accreditation by the Joint Commission

- assists organizations in improving the safety and quality of the care they provide;
- strengthens community confidence;
- provides professional consultation and ongoing support;
- enhances staff education and recruitment;
- fulfills licensure and certification requirements in many states;
- attracts professional referrals;
- conveys Medicare and Medicaid certification for organizations in some accreditation programs; and
- is recognized by insurers, expedites third-party payment, and may favorably influence liability insurance premiums.

Major Initiatives

The Joint Commission works to improve the safety and quality of health care through such projects as the Sentinel Event Database and the ORYX initiative. The former permits dissemination of lessons learned from analysis of serious adverse events by accredited organizations; the latter is establishing performance measurement requirements and supporting quality improvement efforts within accredited organization.

The Joint Commission has also recently launched a Disease-Specific Care certification program. The standards-based program also incorporates the use of clinical practice guidelines and performance measures. Finally, accreditation services for office-based surgery are now being provided under the Ambulatory Care program.

Consumers can gain information on JCAHO-accredited health care organizations on-line through Quality Check™, which is accessible through the Joint Commission's Web site at www.jcaho.org. Performance reports, providing more detailed information about each accredited institution, are also available through Quality Check™.

Origins/Governance

The Joint Commission was founded in 1951. Its governing Board of Commissioners consists of 28 individuals whose experience reflects a broad range of professional and lay interests. The board includes practicing physicians, health care executives, nurses, and public members whose expertise includes bioethics, labor relations, business, insurance, education, and quality improvement, among others. The established reputation of the Joint Commission as a health care quality evaluator permits it direct access to a wide array of experts and public policy makers to guide it in developing and maintaining state-of-the-art standards and performance measures.

Joint Commission on Accreditation of Healthcare
Organizations (JCAHO)
One Renaissance Blvd
Oakbrook Terrace, IL 60181
630 792-5000
630 792-5005 Fax
www.jcaho.org

National Association Medical Staff Services

Formed in 1978, the National Association Medical Staff Services (NAMSS) is an international association that provides professional education resources to individuals in the areas of health care credentialing, clinical privileging, practitioner/provider organizations, and regulatory compliance. Its mission is to protect and promote high-quality health care for the public by helping its members understand and succeed in the changing organizational structures of the health care industry. It also develops, administers, and promotes certification programs that measure knowledge of current industry standards and practices.

For more information, contact:

National Association Medical Staff Services
8317 Cross Park Dr/#150
Austin, TX 78754

Mailing address:
PO Box 140647
Austin, TX 78714-0647

512 454-7928
512 381-6036 Fax
www.namss.org

National Committee for Quality Assurance

The National Committee for Quality Assurance (NCQA) is a private, not-for-profit organization that assesses and reports on the quality of managed care plans, providing a basis for purchasers and consumers of managed health care to distinguish among plans. The efforts of the NCQA are organized around accreditation and performance measurement.

NCQA accreditation surveys are conducted by teams of physicians and managed care experts. A national oversight committee of physicians analyzes the team's findings and assigns one of four possible accreditation levels (full, 1-year, provisional, or denial) based on the plan's level of compliance with NCQA standards.

Origins and Scope

The NCQA began accrediting managed care organizations (MCOs) in 1991 in response to the need for standardized, objective information about the quality of these organizations. Since then, its has expanded the range of organizations that it accredits or certifies to include managed behavioral health care organizations, credentials verification organizations, and physician organizations. More than 75% of all Americans covered by HMOs are in HMOs that have been reviewed by the NCQA.

Accreditation

More than half the HMOs in the nation are currently involved in the NCQA accreditation process. Organizations seeking NCQA accreditation must undergo a survey and meet certain standards designed to evaluate the health plan's clinical and administrative systems, including efforts to continuously improve the quality of care and service it delivers.

During an accreditation survey, plans are reviewed against more than 50 standards, which fall into six categories:

- Quality improvement (40% of a plan's score)
- Physician credentials (20%)
- Members' rights and responsibilities (10%)
- Preventive health services (15%)
- Utilization management (10%)
- Medical records (5%)

Performance Measurement

HEDIS

In addition to examining a health plan's structures and systems through accreditation, the NCQA looks at the results or outcomes the plan actually achieves. It manages the principal performance measurement tool for managed care, the Health Plan Employer Data and Information Set (HEDIS), a set of 71 standardized measures used to evaluate and compare health plans.

Work related to HEDIS has led to projects in distributing performance data, ensuring data accuracy, and making sure the performance data are useful to help guide choice. The NCQA's work in the area of performance measurement focuses on four key areas: HEDIS; NCQA's Quality Compass (a national database of HEDIS data and accreditation information); audit procedures; and consumer research.

Performance Measurement Coordinating Council

To bring consistency to their independent assessment initiatives, NCQA, the Joint Commission on Accreditation of Healthcare Organizations, and the American Medical Accreditation Program have formed the Performance Measurement Coordinating Council, through which they will collaborate to develop and implement coherent and efficient performance measures in health care.

For more information, contact:

National Committee for Quality Assurance
2000 L St NW/Ste 500
Washington, DC 20036
202 955-3500
202 955-3599 Fax
www.ncqa.org

Appendixes

Appendix A

Boards of Medical Examiners in the United States and Possessions

Larry Dixon, Executive Director
Alabama Board of Medical Examiners
848 Washington Ave
Montgomery AL 36104
334 242-4116
334 242-4155 Fax
http://www.albme.org/

Leslie Gallant, Executive Administrator
Alaska State Medical Board
Division of Occupational Licensing
550 W Seventh Ave, Suite 1500
Anchorage AK 99501
907 269-8163
907 269-8196 Fax
http://www.dced.state.ak.us/occ/pmed.htm
E-mail: Leslie_Gallant@dced.state.ak.us

Claudia Foutz, Executive Director
Arizona Board of Medical Examiners
9545 E Doubletree Ranch Rd
Scottsdale AZ 85258
480 551-2700
480 551-2704 Fax
http://www.bomex.org

Peggy Pryor Cryer, Executive Secretary
Arkansas State Medical Board
2100 Riverfront Dr
Little Rock AR 72202-1793
501 296-1802
501 296-1805 Fax
www.armedicalboard.org
E-mail: regdis@armedicalboard.org

Ronald Joseph, Executive Director
Medical Board of California
1426 Howe Ave, Ste 54
Sacramento CA 95825-3236
916 263-2389
916 263-2387
http://www.medbd.ca.gov or http://www.docboard.org

Susan Miller, Program Administrator
Colorado Board of Medical Examiners
1560 Broadway, Ste 1300
Denver CO 80202-5140
303 894-7690
303 894-7692 Fax
http://www.dora.state.co.us/medical
E-mail: susan.miller@dora.state.co.us

Shin-Yu Kettering, Health Program Assistant
State of Connecticut, Department of Public Health
Physician Licensure Unit
PO Box 340308, 410 Capital Ave, MS #12APP
Hartford CT 06134-0308
860 509-7577
860 509-8457 Fax
http://www.state.ct.us/dph/

Gayle Franzolino, Interim Executive Director
Delaware Board of Medical Practice
861 Silver Lake Blvd, Ste 203
Dover DE 19904
302 744-4520
302 739-2711 Fax
E-mail: gfranzolino@state.de.us

James Granger, Executive Director
District of Columbia Board of Medicine
825 North Capitol St NE, Rm 2224
Washington DC 20002
202 442-4777
202 442-9431 Fax
www.dchealth.com

Tanya Williams, Executive Director
Florida Board of Medicine
Bin # C03
4052 Bald Cypress Way
Tallahassee FL 32399
850 245-4131
850 488-9325 Fax
http://www.doh.state.fl.us/mqa
E-mail: Tanya_Williams@doh.state.fl.us

Karen Mason, Executive Director
Georgia Composite State Board of Medical Examiners
2 Peachtree Street, 36th floor
Atlanta GA 30303
404 657-6492
404 656-9723 Fax
http://www.medicalboard.state.ga.us
E-mail: kamason@dch.state.ga.us

Teofilia P Cruz, RN MS, Executive Director
Guam Board of Medical Examiners
1304 E Sunset Blvd
Agana GU 96910-2816
671 475-0251 or 0252
671 477-4733 Fax
E-mail: tcruz@ncsbn.org

Constance Cabral-Makanani, Executive Director
Hawaii Board of Medical Examiners
1010 Richards St
Honolulu HI 96813
808 586-2708
www.state.hi.us

Nancy Kerr, Executive Director
Idaho State Board of Medicine
PO Box 83720
Boise ID 83720-0058
208 327-7000
208 327-7005 Fax
www.bom.state.id.us
E-mail: tsolt@bom.state.id.us

Alicia Purchase, Manager, Medical Unit
Illinois Board of Medical Examiners
Department of Professional Regulation
320 W Washington, 3rd Fl, Med-1
Springfield IL 62786
217 557-3209
217 524-2169 Fax
http://www.dpr.state.il.us/

Angela Smith Jones JD, Board Director
Indiana Health Professions Bureau
402 W Washington St, Rm 041
Indianapolis IN 46204
317 232-2960
317 233-4236 Fax
http://www.ai.org/hpb
E-mail: ajones@hpb.state.in.us

Ann Mowery, PhD, Executive Director
Iowa Board of Medical Examiners
Suite C
400 SW 8th Street
Des Moines IA 50309-4686
515 242-6039
515 242-5908 Fax
http://www.docboard.org/ia/ia_home.htm
E-mail: amowery@ibme.state.ia.us

Lawrence Buening JD, Executive Director
Kansas Board of Healing Arts
235 SW Topeka Blvd
Topeka KS 66603-3068
785 296-3680
785 296-0852 Fax
http://www.ksbha.org/
E-mail: lbuening@ink.org

C. William Schmidt, Executive Director
Kentucky Board of Medical Licensure
310 Whittington Pkwy, Ste 1B
Louisville KY 40222
502 429-8046
502 429-9923 Fax
www.state.ky.us/agencies/kbml

Virginia Benoist JD, Executive Director
Louisiana State Board of Medical Examiners
630 Camp St
New Orleans LA 70130
504 568-6820 x262
504 568-8893 Fax
http://www.lsbme.org

Randal Manning, Executive Director
Maine Board of Licensure in Medicine
137 State House Station
Augusta ME 04333
207 287-3601
207 287-6590 Fax
http://www.docboard.org

C Irving Pinder, Executive Director
Maryland Board of Physician Quality Assurance
PO Box 2571
4201 Patterson Ave, 3rd Fl
Baltimore MD 21215-0095
410 764-4777
410 358-2252 Fax
http://www.docboard.org
E-mail: bpqa@erols.com

Nancy Achin Sullivan, Executive Director
Massachusetts Board of Registration in Medicine
10 West St, 3rd Fl
Boston MA 02111
617 727-3086
617 357-8453 Fax
http://www.docboard.org

Melanie Brim, Director of Licensing, Bureau of Health
Services
Michigan Board of Medicine
611 W Ottawa St
Lansing MI 48933
517 373-6873
517 241-3082 Fax
http://www.cis.state.mi.us/bhser
E-mail: mbbrim@michigan.gov

Robert Leach, JD, Executive Director
Minnesota Board of Medical Practice
University Park Plaza
2829 University Ave SE, Ste 400
Minneapolis MN 55414-3246
612 617-2130
612 617-2166 Fax
http://www.bmp.state.mn.us

W Joseph Burnett MD, Director
Mississippi State Board of Medical Licensure
1867 Crane Ridge Dr, Ste 200B
Jackson MS 39216
601 987-3079
601 987-4159 Fax
http://www.msbml.state.ms.us
E-mail: mboard@msbml.state.ms.us

Tina Steinman, Executive Director
**Missouri State Board of Registration for
the Healing Arts**
Division of Professional Registration
3605 Missouri Blvd
Jefferson City MO 65109
573 751-0098
573 751-3166 Fax
http://www.ecodev.state.mo.us/pr/healarts
E-mail: tsteinma@mail.state.mo.us

Jeannie Worsech, Executive Director
Montana Board of Medical Examiners
PO Box 200513
301 S Park Ave, 4th Floor
Helena MT 59620-0513
406 841-2360
406 841-2363 Fax
http://commerce.state.mt.us/POLMain/index.html

Becky Wisell, Executive Director
Nebraska Health and Human Services System
Department of Regulation and Licensure,
Credentialing Division
301 Centennial Mall South, PO Box 94986
Lincoln NE 68509-4986
402 471-2118
402 471-3577 Fax
http://www.hhs.state.ne.us
E-mail: becky.wisell@hhs.state.ne.us

Larry Lessly, JD, Executive Director
Nevada State Board of Medical Examiners
Ste 301
1105 Terminal Way
Reno NV 89502
775 688-2559
775 688-2321 Fax
http://www.state.nv.us/medical
E-mail: nsbme@govmail.state.nv.us

Penny Taylor, Administrator
New Hampshire Board of Medicine
2 Industrial Park Dr, Ste 8
Concord NH 03301-8520
603 271-1204
603 271-6702 Fax
http://www.state.nh.us/medicine
E-mail: ptaylor@nhsa.state.nh.us

William Roeder, Executive Director
New Jersey State Board of Medical Examiners
PO Box 183
140 E Front Street, 2nd FL
Trenton NJ 08625-0183
609 826-7100
609 777-0956 Fax
http://www.state.nj.us

Charlotte Kinney, Executive Director
New Mexico Board of Medical Examiners
Lamy Bldg, 2nd Fl
491 Old Santa Fe Trail
Santa Fe NM 87501
505 827-7363
505 827-7377 Fax
E-mail: charlotte.kinney@state.nm.us

Thomas Monahan, Executive Secretary
New York State Education Department
Cultural Education Center, Rm 3023
Empire State Plaza
Albany NY 12230
518 474-3817 x340
518 486-4846 Fax
http://www.op.nysed.gov
E-mail: tmonahan@mail.nysed.gov

Andy Watry, Executive Director
North Carolina Medical Board
1201 Front St
Raleigh NC 27609
919 326-1100 ext 221
919 326-1130 or 326-1131 Fax
www.ncmedboard.org
E-mail: info@ncmedboard.org

Rolf Sletten, JD, Executive Secretary and Treasurer
North Dakota State Board of Medical Examiners
418 E Broadway Ave, Ste 12
Bismarck ND 58501
701 328-6500
701 328-6505 Fax
http://www.ndbomex.com
E-mail: bomex@tic.bisman.com

Thomas Dilling, Executive Director
State Medical Board of Ohio
77 S High St, 17th Fl
Columbus OH 43215
614 466-3934
614 728-5946 Fax
http://www.state.oh.us/med
E-mail: Tom.Dilling@med.state.oh.us

Lyle Kelsey, Executive Director
Oklahoma Board of Medical Licensure and Supervision
PO Box 18256
Oklahoma City OK 73154-0256
405 848-6841
405 848-8240 Fax
http://www.osbmls.state.ok.us
E-mail: lkelsey@osbmls.state.ok.us

Kathleen Haley JD, Executive Director
Oregon Board of Medical Examiners
620 Crown Plaza
1500 SW First Ave
Portland OR 97201-5826
503 229-5770
503 229-6543
www.bme.state.or.us/

Cindy Warner, Administrative Officer
Pennsylvania State Board of Medicine
116 Pine St
Harrisburg PA 17101
717 787-2381
717 787-7769 Fax
www.dos.state.pa.us

Ivonne Fernandez Colon, Executive Director
Puerto Rico Board of Medical Examiners
Department of Health
PO Box 13969
San Juan PR 00908
787 782-8949 or 782-8937
787 792-4436 Fax

Milton Hamolsky, MD, Chief Administrative Officer
**Rhode Island Board of Medical Licensure
and Discipline**
Joseph E Cannon Bldg, Rm 205
Three Capitol Hill
Providence RI 02908-5097
401 222-3855
401 222-2158 Fax
http://www.docboard.org/ri/main.htm

John Volmer, Interim Board Administrator
**South Carolina Department of Labor, Licensing &
Regulation**
PO Box 11289
110 Centerview Dr, Ste 202
Columbia SC 29211-1289
803 896-4500
803 896-4515 Fax
http://www.llr.sc.us/
E-mail: medboard@zip.llr.sc.edu

L Paul Jensen, Executive Secretary
**South Dakota State Board of Medical & Osteopathic
Examiners**
1323 S Minnesota Ave
Sioux Falls SD 57105
605 334-8343
605 336-0270 Fax

Rosemarie Otto, Executive Director
Tennessee Department of Health
First Floor, Cordell Hull Bldg
425 5th Avenue North
Nashville TN 37247-1010
615 741-4540
615 253-4484 Fax
http://www.state.tn.us/health
E-mail: rosemarie.otto@mail.state.tn.us

Jerry Walker, Interim Executive Director
Texas State Board of Medical Examiners
PO Box 2018
Austin TX 78768-2018
512 305-7010
512 305-7006 Fax
http://www.tsbme.state.tx.us or
http://www.docboard.org/aim.htm

Diana Baker, MSN RNC
State of Utah Department of Commerce
Division of Occupational & Professional Licensing
PO Box 146741, 160 East 300 South
Salt Lake City UT 84114-6741
801 530-6179
801 530-6511 Fax
http://www.commerce.state.ut.us
E-mail: dbaker@utah.gov

Lydia Scott, Executive Assistant
Virgin Islands Board of Medical Examiners
Office of the Commissioner, Department of Health
48 Sugar Estate
St Thomas VI 00802
340 774-0117
340 777-4001 Fax

William Harp, MD, Executive Director
Virginia Board of Medicine
6606 W Broad St, 4th Fl
Richmond VA 23230-1717
804 662-9960
804 662-9517 Fax
http://www.dhp.state.va.us
E-mail: medbd@dhp.state.va.us

Gloria Hurd, Executive Director
Vermont Board of Medical Practice
109 State St
Montpelier VT 05609-1106
802 828-2818
802 828-5450 Fax
http://www.sec.state.vt.us
E-mail: gloria.hurd@medbd.state.vt.us

Doron Manice, Executive Director
Washington State Department of Public Health
Medical Quality Assurance Commission
PO Box 47866
Olympia WA 98504-7866
360 236-4823
360 586-4573 Fax
http://www.doh.wa.gov/Medical/default.htm
E-mail: doran.maniece@doh.wa.gov

Ronald Walton, Executive Director
West Virginia Board of Medicine
101 Dee Dr
Charleston WV 25311
304 558-2921 x227
304 558-2084 Fax
www.wvdhhr.org/wvbom
E-mail: RonaldWalton@wvdhhr.org

Deanna Zychowski, Bureau Director
State of Wisconsin Medical Examining Board
Bureau of Health Professions, Dept of Regulation & Licensing
1400 E Washington Ave
Madison WI 53703
608 266-5432
608 267-1803 Fax
http://www.wisconsin.gov/state/home
E-mail: deanna.zychowski@drl.state.wi.us

Carole Shotwell, JD, Executive Secretary
Wyoming Board of Medicine
Colony Bldg, 2nd Fl
211 W 19th St
Cheyenne WY 82002
307 778-7053
307 778-2069 Fax
E-mail: wyobom@aol.com

Appendix B

Boards of Osteopathic Medical Examiners in the United States and Possessions

Joyce M Kossick, RPh, Acting Executive Director
Arizona Board of Osteopathic Examiners in Medicine & Surgery
9535 E Doubletree Ranch Rd
Scottsdale AZ 85258
480 657-7703 x29
480 657-7715 Fax
www.azosteoboard.org/home.htm

Linda Bergmann, Executive Director
Osteopathic Medical Board of California
2720 Gateway Oaks Dr, Ste 350
Sacramento CA 95833-3500
916 263-3100
916 263-3117 Fax
www.docboard.org
E-mail: linda_bergmann@dca.ca.gov

Karen Eaton, Executive Director
Florida Board of Osteopathic Medicine
Bin #C06
4052 Bald Cypress Way
Tallahassee FL 32399-3256
850 488-0595
850 487-9874 Fax
http://www.doh.state.fl.us/mqa
E-mail: christy_robinson@doh.state.fl.us

Susan Strout, Executive Secretary
Maine Board of Osteopathic Licensure
142 State House Station
Augusta ME 04333
207 287-2480
207 287-3015 Fax
www.docboard.org/me-osteo
E-mail: susan.e.strout@state.me.us

Melanie Brim, Director of Licensing
Michigan Board of Osteopathic Medicine & Surgery
611 W Ottawa St
Lansing MI 48933
517 373-6873
517 241-3082 Fax
E-mail: mbbrim@michigan.gov

Larry Tarno, DO, Executive Director
Nevada State Board of Osteopathic Medicine
2860 E Flamingo Rd, Ste G
Las Vegas NV 89121
702 732-2147
702 732-2079 Fax

Elizabeth Montoya, Executive Director
New Mexico Board of Osteopathic Medical Examiners
Ste 400
2055 S Pacheco St
Santa Fe NM 87504
505 476-7120
505 476-7095 Fax
www.rld.state.nm.us/b&c/osteopathic_examiners_board.htm
E-mail: osteoboard@state.nm.us

Gary Clark, Executive Director
Oklahoma Board of Osteopathic Examiners
4848 N Lincoln Blvd, Ste 100
Oklahoma City OK 73105-3321
405 528-8625
405 557-0653 Fax
www.docboard.org

Gina Bittner, Administrative Assistant
Pennsylvania State Board of Osteopathic Medicine
PO Box 2649, 116 Pine St
Harrisburg PA 17101
717 783-4858
717 787-7769 Fax
E-mail: gbittner@state.pa.us

Rosemarie Otto, Executive Director
Tennessee State Board of Osteopathic Examiners
First Floor Cordell Hull Bldg
425 5th Avenue North
Nashville TN 37247-1010
615 751-4540
615 532-5164
http://www.state.tn.us/health
E-mail: rosemarie.otto@mail.state.tn.us

Peggy Atkins, Staff Secretary
**Vermont Board of Osteopathic Physicians
and Surgeons**
Vermont Section of State Office, Office of Professional
Regulations
26 Terrace Street, Drawer 09
Montpelier VT 05602-1106
802 828-2373
802 828-2465 Fax
http://www.sec.state.vt.us
E-mail: patkins@sec.state.vt.us

Arlene Robertson, Program Manager
Washington Board of Osteopathic Medicine & Surgery
Department of Health
PO Box 47870
Olympia WA 98504-7870
360 236-4945
360 586-0745 Fax
http://www.doh.wa.gov/hsqa/hpqad/Osteopath/default.htm
E-mail: arlene.robertson@doh.wa.gov

Cheryl Schreiber, Executive Secretary
West Virginia Board of Osteopathy
334 Penco Rd
Weirton WV 26062
304 723-4638
304 723-6723 Fax

Appendix C

Member Boards of the Federation of Medical Licensing Authorities of Canada

Sylvia Smith, Executive Secretary
Federation of Medical Licensing Authorities of Canada
2283 St Laurent Blvd, PO Box 8234
Ottawa, ON K1G 3H7
613 738-0372
613 738-8977 Fax
www.mcc.ca/fmlac/

Robert Burns, MD, Registrar
College of Physicians and Surgeons of Alberta
900 Manulife Place, 10180-101 St
Edmonton, AB T5J 4P8
780 423-4764
780 420-0651 Fax
www.cpsa.ab.ca

Morris Vanandel, MD, Registrar
College of Physicians & Surgeons of British Columbia
1807 W 10th Ave
Vancouver, BC V6J 2A9
604 733-7758
604 733-1047 Fax
www.cpsbc.bc.ca

William Pope, MD, Registrar
College of Physicians and Surgeons of Manitoba
1000-1661 Portage Ave
Winnipeg, MB R3J 3T7
204 774-4344
204 774-0750 Fax
www.umanitoba.ca/colleges/cps

Edmund Schollenberg, MD, Registrar
College of Physicians and Surgeons of New Brunswick
One Hampton Rd, Ste 300
Rothesay, NB E2E 5K8
506 849-5050
506 849-5069 Fax
www.cpsnb.org

Robert W. Young, MD, Registrar
Newfoundland Medical Board
139 Water St, St John's, NF A1C 1B2
709 726-8546
709 726-4725 Fax
E-mail: nbm@thezone.net

Cameron Little, MD, Registrar
College of Physicians and Surgeons of Nova Scotia
200-1559 Brunswick St, Sentry Place
Halifax, NS B3J 2G1
902 422-5823
902 422-5035 Fax
www.cpsns.ns.ca

Jeannette Hall, Registrar
Department of Health and Social Service
Government of the Northwest Territories
Centre Square Tower
5022 49th St, 8th Fl, PO Box 1320
Yellowknife, NWT X1A 2L9
867 920-8058
867 873-0281 Fax
E-mail: jeannette_hall@gov.nt.ca

Rocco Gerace, MD, Registrar
College of Physicians and Surgeons of Ontario
80 College St
Toronto, ON M5G 2E2
416 967-2600 or 800 268-7096
416 961-3330 Fax
www.cpso.on.ca

Cyril Moyse, MD, Registrar
College of Physicians and Surgeons of
Prince Edward Island
199 Grafton St
Charlottetown, PEI C1A 1L2
902 566-3861
902 566-3861 Fax
E-mail: moyfive@atcon.com

Joelle Lescop, MD, Secrétaire-générale
College des médecins du Québec
2170 boul René Lévésque ouest
Montréal, PQ H3H 2T8
514 933-4441
514 933-3112 Fax
www.cmq.org

Dennis A. Kendel, MD, Registrar
College of Physicians and Surgeons of Saskatchewan
211 4th Ave S
Saskatoon, SK S7K 1N1
306 244-7355
306 244-0090 Fax
www.quadrant.net/cpss

Elsie Bagan, Registrar
Department of Consumer and Corporate Affairs
Government of the Yukon
2130 Second Ave, 3rd Floor
PO Box 2703
Whitehorse, YT Y1A 2C6
867 667-5257
867 667-3609 Fax
E-mail: elsie.bagan@gov.yk.ca

Appendix D

Glossary of Medical Licensure Terms and List of Common Abbreviations

Common Abbreviations

ABMS	American Board of Medical Specialties
ACGME	Accreditation Council for Graduate Medical Education
AMA PRA	American Medical Association Physician's Recognition Award
AOA	American Osteopathic Association
CME	Continuing medical education
COMLEX	Comprehensive Osteopathic Medical Licensing Examination
COMVEX	Comprehensive Osteopathic Medical Variable Purpose Examination
ECFMG	Educational Commission for Foreign Medical Graduates
FCVS	Federation Credentials Verification Service
FLEX	Federation Licensing Examination
FSMB	Federation of State Medical Boards
FWA	Federation Licensing Examination (FLEX) Weighted Average
GMC	Graduate Medical Council (United Kingdom)
GME	Graduate medical education
IMG	International medical graduate
JCAHO	Joint Commission on Accreditation of Healthcare Organizations
LCME	Liaison Committee on Medical Education
LMCC	Licentiate of the Medical Council of Canada
NAMSS	National Association Medical Staff Services
NBME	National Board of Medical Examiners
NBOME	National Board of Osteopathic Medical Examiners
NCQA	National Committee for Quality Assurance
PRA	American Medical Association Physician's Recognition Award
SBE	State board examination
SPEX	Special Purpose Examination
USMLE	United States Medical Licensing Examination
VQE	Visa Qualifying Examination

Definitions

Accreditation Council for Graduate Medical Education (ACGME)

An accrediting agency with five member organizations:

- American Board of Medical Specialties
- American Hospital Association
- American Medical Association
- Association of American Medical Colleges
- Council of Medical Specialty Societies

Each member organization nominates four directors. The federal government names a representative to serve in a nonvoting capacity, and the ACGME chooses three public representatives. There is also a resident representative, and the chair of the Residency Review Committee Council sits as a voting representative. The mission of the ACGME is to improve the quality of health in the United States by ensuring and improving the quality of allopathic graduate medical education experience for physicians in training. The ACGME establishes national standards for graduate medical education by which it approves and continually assesses educational programs under its aegis. The ACGME accredits GME programs through its 27 review committees (26 Residency Review Committees, or RRCs, and the Transitional Year Review Committee).

American Board of Medical Specialties (ABMS)

A nonprofit organization of 24 approved medical specialty boards. Its mission is to maintain and improve the quality of medical care by helping its member boards develop and use professional and educational standards for the evaluation and certification of physician specialists. The certification of physicians provides assurance to the public that a physician specialist certified by an ABMS member board has successfully completed an approved educational program and an evaluation process that assesses the knowledge, skills, and experience required to provide quality patient care in that specialty. Medical specialty board certification is an additional process to receiving a medical degree, completing residency training, and receiving a license to practice medicine.

Certification

A voluntary process intended to assure the public that a certified medical specialist has successfully completed an approved educational program and an evaluation including an examination process designed to assess the knowledge, experience, and skills requisite to the provision of high-quality patient care in that specialty.

Clerkship

Clinical education provided to medical students. Table 9 on p. 30 contains information on clerkship regulations of state medical boards.

Clinical Skills Assessment (CSA)

A 1-day exam that requires examinees to demonstrate both clinical proficiency and spoken English language proficiency. The CSA is administered throughout the year at the ECFMG Clinical Skills Assessment Center in Philadelphia, Pennsylvania.

Comprehensive Osteopathic Medical Licensing Examination (COMLEX-USA)

A three-level examination initiated in 1995 by the National Board of Osteopathic Medical Examiners to replace the former three-part NBOME examination series and to better assist the state licensing boards in measuring the knowledge required by today's physicians.

The COMLEX-USA program is designed to assess the osteopathic medical knowledge considered essential for osteopathic generalist physicians to practice medicine without supervision. COMLEX is constructed in the context of medical problem solving, which involves clinical presentations and physician tasks.

Educational Commission for Foreign Medical Graduates (ECFMG)

A nonprofit organization that assesses the readiness of graduates of foreign medical schools to enter residency programs in the United States accredited by the Accreditation Council for Graduate Medical Education (ACGME).

ECFMG certification provides assurance to directors of ACGME-accredited residency programs, and to the people of the United States, that graduates of foreign medical schools have met minimum standards of eligibility required to enter such programs. This certification does not guarantee that such graduates will be accepted into these programs in the United States, since the number of applicants frequently exceeds the number of positions available.

ECFMG certification is also a prerequisite required by most states for licensure to practice medicine in the United States and is one of the eligibility requirements to take Step 3 of the United States Medical Licensing Examination (USMLE).

ECFMG number

The number assigned by the Educational Commission for Foreign Medical Graduates (ECFMG) to each international medical graduate (IMG) who applies for certification from ECFMG. Almost all graduates of foreign medical schools must have an ECFMG certificate to participate in graduate medical education in the United States.

Endorsement, licensure

A process through which a state issues an unrestricted license to practice medicine to an individual who holds a valid and unrestricted license in another jurisdiction. Licensure endorsement is generally based on documentation of successfully completing approved examinations, authentication of required core documents, and completion of any additional requirements assessing the applicant's fitness to practice medicine in the new jurisdiction. Previously referred to as "reciprocity."

Fellow

A. A physician in an ACGME-accredited program that is beyond the requirements for eligibility for first board certification in the discipline. Such physicians may also be termed "resident" as well. Other uses of the term "fellow" require modifiers for precision and clarity, eg, "research fellow." *Also see "Resident or resident physician."*

B. A physician who has demonstrated outstanding achievements in medicine, usually within a given medical specialty society. Typical criteria for fellowship in a specialty society include years of membership, years as a practitioner in the specialty, and professional recognition by peers.

Fifth Pathway

One of several ways that individuals who obtain their undergraduate medical education abroad can enter GME in the United States. The Fifth Pathway is a period of supervised clinical training for students who obtained their premedical education in the United States, received undergraduate medical education abroad, and passed Step 1 of the United States Medical Licensing Examination. After these students successfully complete a year of clinical training sponsored by a US medical school accredited by the Liaison Committee on Medical Education (LCME) and pass USMLE Step 2, they receive a Fifth Pathway certificate and become eligible for an ACGME-accredited residency as an international medical graduate. Currently, New York Medical College in Valhalla, New York is the primary medical school that offers the Fifth Pathway.

Federation Licensing Examination (FLEX)

Originally introduced in 1968 and subsequently enhanced and modified in 1985, this examination was administered for the last time in December 1993. In 1994, the United States Medical Licensing Examination (USMLE) was fully implemented. Some candidates for licensure may have a combination of scores from FLEX and USMLE. *Also see "United States Medical Licensing Examination."*

Federation of State Medical Boards (FSMB)

A nonprofit organization whose membership comprises the 70 allopathic, osteopathic, and composite medical licensing boards of all the states, the District of Columbia, Guam, Puerto Rico, and the Virgin Islands. Its primary responsibility is to protect the public through the regulation of physicians and other health care providers. It serves as a liaison, advocate, and information source to the public, health care organizations, and state, national, and international authorities. The FSMB promotes high standards for physician licensure and practice and assists and supports state medical boards collectively and individually in the regulation of medical practice and in their role of public protection.

FLEX Weighted Average (FWA)

All states currently require a minimum passing score of 75 on each component of the post-1985 two-part FLEX; the resulting number composes the Federation Licensing Examination (FLEX) Weighted Average.

Intern

No longer used by the AMA or ACGME. Historically, "intern" was used to designate individuals in the first post-MD year of hospital training; less commonly, it designated individuals in the first year of any residency program. Since 1975, the AMA's *Graduate Medical Education Directory* and the ACGME have used "resident," "resident physician," or "fellow" to designate all individuals in ACGME-accredited programs. *Also see "Resident or resident physician" and "Fellow."*

International medical graduate (IMG)

A graduate from a medical school outside the US and Canada. Formerly referred to as "foreign medical graduate" (FMG).

Initial license

The first ever full and unrestricted license a physician receives in his/her medical career. Some medical boards interpret "initial license" as a physician's first license in their particular states (although the physician could already have been licensed in other states). This publication does not use the term in this sense.

Liaison Committee on Medical Education (LCME)

The body that accredits educational programs in the US and Canada leading to the MD degree. The American Osteopathic Association (AOA) accredits educational programs leading to the doctor of osteopathy (DO) degree.

Licensure

The process by which a state or jurisdiction of the United States admits physicians to the practice of medicine. Licensure ensures that practicing physicians have appropriate education and training and that they abide by recognized standards of professional conduct while serving their patients. Candidates for first licensure must complete a rigorous examination designed to assess a physician's ability to apply knowledge, concepts, and principles that are important in health and disease and that constitute the basis of safe and effective patient care. All applicants must submit proof of medical education and training and provide details about their work history. Finally, applicants may have to reveal information regarding past medical history (including the use of habit-forming drugs and emotional or mental illness), arrests, and convictions. *Also see "Limited license" and "Reregistration."*

Limited license

Issued by state medical boards to resident physicians in graduate medical education (GME) programs within their jurisdictions. Physicians do not receive a full and unrestricted license until completion of GME and fulfillment of other licensure requirements in a given jurisdiction.

Locum tenens

This Latin term (locum "place," tenens "to hold") describes a person taking another's place for the time being. In medicine, for example, the American Medical Association's Project USA provides short-term replacements for US Public Health Service physicians in rural locations, allowing them to take a vacation or fulfill continuing medical education requirements (see "Project USA," p. 111).

Medical Practice Act

A statute of a US state or jurisdiction that outlines the practice of medicine and the responsibility of the medical board to regulate that practice. The primary responsibility and obligation of a state medical board is to protect the public through proper licensing and regulation of physicians and, in some jurisdictions, other health care professionals. *Also see "Unprofessional conduct."*

National Board of Medical Examiners (NBME)

A nonprofit, independent organization that prepares and administers medical qualifying examinations, either independently or jointly with other organizations. Legal agencies governing the practice of medicine within each US state or jurisdiction may grant a license without further examination for those physicians who have successfully completed such examinations and met other requirements.

Currently, the NBME administers USMLE Steps 1 and 2 to students and graduates of US and Canadian medical and osteopathic schools accredited by the Liaison Committee on Medical Education or the American Osteopathic Association.

National Board of Osteopathic Medical Examiners (NBOME)

A not-for-profit corporation serving the public and state licensing agencies by administering examinations testing the medical knowledge of those who seek to practice as osteopathic physicians.

The NBOME examinations have been the primary pathway by which osteopathic physicians have applied for licensure to practice osteopathic medicine. A passing score on these examinations verifies a student's adequacy of medical knowledge for practicing osteopathic medicine.

Reregistration

After physicians are licensed in a state or jurisdiction, they must reregister periodically to continue their active status. During this reregistration process, physicians are required to demonstrate that they have maintained acceptable standards of ethics and medical practice and have not engaged in improper conduct. In some states, physicians must also show that they have participated in a program of continuing medical education.

Resident or resident physician

Any individual at any level in an ACGME-accredited GME program, including subspecialty programs. Local usage might refer to these individuals as interns, house officers, house staff, trainees, fellows, or other comparable terminology. Beginning in 2000, the ACGME has used the term "fellow" to denote physicians in subspecialty programs (versus residents in specialty programs) or in GME programs that are beyond the requirements for eligibility for first board certification in the discipline. *Also see "Fellow."*

Special Purpose Examination (SPEX)

This 1-day, computer-administered examination, with approximately 420 multiple-choice questions, assesses primary care medical knowledge and skills. It does not include questions specific to a particular specialty or subspecialty. The SPEX is used to assess physicians who have held a valid, unrestricted license in a US or Canadian jurisdiction who are:

- required by the state medical board to demonstrate current medical knowledge,
- seeking endorsement licensure some years beyond initial examination, or
- seeking license reinstatement after a period of professional inactivity.

Physicians holding a valid, unrestricted license may also apply for SPEX, independent of any request or approval from a medical licensing board.

Telemedicine

Telemedicine is the delivery of health care services via electronic means from a health care provider in one location to a patient in another. Applications that fall under this definition include the transfer of medical images, such as pathology slides or radiographs, interactive video consultations between patient and provider or between primary care and specialty care physicians, and mental health consultations (see Table 17 for more information).

Unprofessional conduct

Although laws vary from one jurisdiction to the next, the Medical Practice Acts in force in most US jurisdictions would define unprofessional conduct as including:

- physical abuse of a patient
- inadequate recordkeeping
- not recognizing or acting on common symptoms
- prescribing drugs in excessive amounts or without legitimate reason
- impaired ability to practice due to addiction or physical or mental illness
- failing to meet continuing medical education requirements
- performing duties beyond the scope of a license
- dishonesty
- conviction of a felony
- delegating the practice of medicine to an unlicensed individual

Unprofessional conduct would not include minor disagreements or poor customer service.

United States Medical Licensing Examination (USMLE)

This 3-step examination for US medical licensure provides a common evaluation system for applicants. The USMLE program is governed by a composite committee of representatives from the Federation of State Medical Boards (FSMB), the National Board of Medical Examiners (NBME), the Educational Commission for Foreign Medical Graduates (ECFMG), and the public.

Results of the USMLE are reported to state medical boards for use in granting the initial license to practice medicine. Each medical licensing authority requires, as part of its licensing processes, successful completion of an examination or other certification demonstrating qualification for licensure.

The USMLE replaced FLEX and the certifying examination of the NBME, as well as the Foreign Medical Graduate Examination in the Medical Sciences (FMGEMS), which was formerly used by the ECFMG for certification purposes. Steps 1 and 2 of the USMLE are used as the examination for ECFMG certification. These two steps are also used for promotion and graduation in some US medical schools.

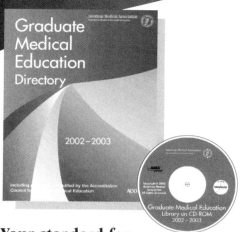
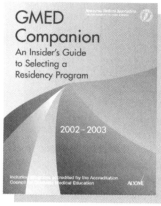